INTERMEDIATE EMERGENCY CARE EXAM REVIEW

Richard A. Cherry
Clinical Instructor
Director of Paramedic Training
Department of Emergency Medicine
SUNY Health Science Center
Syracuse, New York

BRADY
Prentice Hall
Upper Saddle River, New Jersey 07458

Library of Congress Cataloging-in-Publication Data

Cherry, Richard A.
 Intermediate emergency care exam review / Richard A. Cherry.
  p. cm.
 ISBN 0-8359-4978-8
  1. Emergency medicine—Examinations, questions, etc. 2. Emergency medical technicians
 —Examinations, questions, etc. I. Title.
  [DNLM: 1. Emergencies—examination questions. 2. Emergency Medical Services
 —examination questions. 3. Emergency Medical Technicians—examination questions. WB 18.2
 C522i 1996]
 RC86.9.C438 1996
 616.02'5'076—dc20
 DNLM/DLC
 for Library of Congress   95-33565
                                                                                                                      CIP

Publisher: Susan Katz
Managing Production Editor: Patrick Walsh
Copy Editor: Rose Kernan
Manufacturing Buyer: Ilene Sanford
Page Layout: Stephen Hartner

 © 1996 by Prentice-Hall, Inc.
A Simon & Schuster Company
Upper Saddle River, NJ 07458

All rights reserved. No part of this book may be
reproduced, in any form or by any means,
without permission in writing from the publisher.

Printed in the United State of America
10 9 8 7 6 5 4 3 2 1

ISBN 0-8359-4978-8

PRENTICE-HALL INTERNATIONAL (UK) LIMITED, *London*
PRENTICE-HALL OF AUSTRALIA PTY. LIMITED, *Sydney*
PRENTICE-HALL CANADA INC., *Toronto*
Prentice-Hall Hispanoamericano, S.A., *Mexico*
PRENTICE-HALL OF INDIA PRIVATE LIMITED, *New Delhi*
PRENTICE-HALL OF JAPAN, INC., *Tokyo*
SIMON & SCHUSTER ASIA PTE. LTD., *Singapore*
EDITORA PRENTICE-HALL DO BRASIL, LTDA., *Rio de Janeiro*

To my big brother, Bill,
who has provided me with inspiration,
a conservative viewpoint,
and comic relief
when I needed it most.

Contents

To the Student, vii

Chapter 1   Roles and Responsibilities of the EMT-Intermediate, 1

Chapter 2   Emergency Medical Services Systems, 5

Chapter 3   Medical Legal Considerations in Emergency Care, 11

Chapter 4   Medical Terminology, 17

Chapter 5   EMS Communications, 25

Chapter 6   General Patient Assessment and Initial Management, 30

Chapter 7   Advanced Airway Management and Ventilation, 39

Chapter 8   Fluids and Shock, 52

Appendices   Defibrillation, Blood Glucose Determination, Administration of 50% Glucose, Subcutaneous Medication Administration, Intramuscular Medication Administration, Administration of Nebulized Medications, Accessing Indwelling Catheters, Pulse Oximetry, 66

To the Student

The future belongs to those who believe in the beauty of their dreams.

Eleanor Roosevelt

This book is designed to help you prepare for both your certification exams and for the streets. I have provided for you over 300 multiple choice questions covering every chapter of *Intermediate Emergency Care* (IEC) and the USDOT Intermediate Curriculum. The questions test your knowledge, your understanding, and your ability to apply your knowledge in emergency medical scenarios. I also have provided the correct answer to each question, the rationale for the answer, and the page number from *Intermediate Emergency Care* where you will find a more detailed explanation. The final ingredient is desire, which you must provide.

The great American poet, Henry David Thoreau, once wrote, "If one advances confidently in the direction of his dreams and endeavors to live the life which he has imagined, he will meet with a success unexpected in common hours." *Kaizen* is a Japanese word that means making a lifelong commitment toward self-improvement. This Oriental philosophy encourages life satisfaction through continual personal and professional growth. It is a never-ending process of making small, incremental improvements in your life. If there was ever a group of people who should adopt the Kaizen philosophy in their lives, it's EMS providers. Turning your professional life into an endless quest for perfection brings with it a measure of success. It is the journey—not the goal—that enriches our lives. It's like taking a cruise. The object is not to get to your destination as quickly as possible but to have fun getting there. Likewise, success is not a destination, but a journey. When you make this commitment, you begin to reap the rewards immediately. The moment you set sail on this course, you and your future patients benefit from your increased commitment. Providing emergency medical care is a tremendous privilege. With this privilege comes the responsibility to do your very best academic work. Think about how much patient care you will affect. Think about how many people's lives you will influence. Do so and you should begin to realize the tremendous responsibility you accept when you bear the title of "EMS provider"!

The formula is simple. Turn your weaknesses into your strengths. The first step is to identify your weak areas. This step is difficult, but critical. It's not easy because you must admit that you're not doing the job you could be doing. It's much easier to become complacent about your abilities. It's much easier to become comfortable with your present performance and accept your limitations as such. The consequences of this kind of attitude, however, are alarming. Patients suffer from your lack of knowledge and skill. Use this book of questions to identify your weak areas.

Once you have identified your weaknesses make the personal commitment to improve in those areas. World-class athletes measure improvements by fractions of seconds and inches. They work tirelessly on making tiny improvements in the many aspects of their sport. They call it "personal best." You can achieve *your* personal best each year by making small incremental improvements in the needed areas. By improving just one aspect of your craft each year, you make great strides. The short-term results are immediate—you enjoy EMS more because you are becoming better at it. We all enjoy doing the things that we do well. The long-term result is a rewarding career caring for those who are sick or injured.

Former Green Bay Packer football coach Vince Lombardi best described this attitude when he wrote, "Making the effort to be perfect is what life is all about. If you will not settle for anything less than the best, you will be amazed at what you can do with your lives. Winning isn't everything, but making the effort to win is. The difference between a successful person and an unsuccessful one is not a lack of knowledge, or a lack of strength, but a lack of will."

Remember, this is a lifelong journey. Don't try to do it all by Friday, but never give up your quest. You build a successful life one day at a time. Someone once asked Miami Dolphin football coach Don Shula if it wasn't a waste of time trying to correct such a small flaw in his team's offense. Don's reply was "What's a small flaw?" That's striving for perfection. That's a commitment to excellence. That's Kaizen. It's no wonder that his 1972 squad is still the only team ever to complete a perfect season. It's also no wonder that he is the winningest coach in professional football history.

Why make learning a lifelong endeavor? American humorist Will Rogers once said, "Even if you are on the right track, you'll get run over if you just stand there." He was right. I don't believe in the status quo. Either you're getting better or you're getting worse. It's like walking up a down escalator. If you keep moving forward, you'll eventually end up on top. You will at least stay in place. Once you slow down or stop, however, you begin to move downwards until you eventually reach the bottom. A field provider who fails to keep pace with the fast-moving world of emergency medicine soon becomes obsolete, even dangerous. This book is designed to help you maintain a high level of medical knowledge.

The road to excellence is not easy. It's easier to take the path of least resistance. It's easier to back away from excellence than it is to give everything you've got. While it's easier to let frustrations, distractions, and fatigue erode your performance, it's not satisfying in the long run. Making this commitment takes a tremendous amount of courage. If you fail, there are no excuses. You can look yourself in the mirror and know that you gave it your very best. In that effort, you have not failed. When your EMT career is over, you want to look back with no regrets.

Do you want to be great? Many talk the talk, few walk the walk. Many want to be great, but few are willing to pay the price. What is "average"? According to Notre Dame football coach Lou Holtz, "It's the best of the worst or the worst of the best. It's the top of the bottom or the bottom of the top. It's nowhere." Challenge yourself to make a commitment to excellence. If you believe in yourself, you can be as great as you want to be. You must have the courage, the determination, the dedication, and the competitive drive to do it. You must be willing to sacrifice the little things in life and pay the price for the things that are worthwhile. If you can do all these things, great things can happen.

Once you have made a commitment to a way of life, you put the greatest strength in the world behind you. We call it "heart." Once you have made this commitment, nothing will stop you short of success. You have to want to. You have to have a raging desire to be the best you can be. It's not a part-time thing. Athletes call it "competitive anger," and many use this motivational factor to spur them on to greatness. There have been few successful people that didn't have competitive anger driving their talents to the surface. Hall of Fame baseball player Ted Williams once said, "I wanted to be the greatest hitter who ever lived. A man has to have goals—for a day, for a lifetime—and that was mine, to have people say, 'There goes Ted Williams, the greatest hitter who ever lived.'" He was the greatest hitter because he made an unwavering commitment to excellence.

To succeed, you don't have to be the most experienced or the most talented, just the most tenacious. You must hold on to your goals and dreams. Your rewards for making a commitment to excellence cannot be measured financially. You will have the feeling of confidence and self-worth from having accomplished something for yourself. This feeling will transfer into other areas of your life in more ways than you can ever imagine.

The essence of Kaizen is adopting a positive attitude about everything you do. According to this philosophy, attitude is the most important thing you can develop in your life. While ability determines capability, attitude determines performance. You were born with certain abilities. Your attitude determines how close you come to realizing your full potential. Don't dwell on your shortcomings and limitations. Try to work around them. My father used to tell me that things turn out the best for those who make the best out of the way things turn out. Turn your weaknesses into strengths, then measure yourself not by what you have done, but by what you have done with your ability.

You don't have to be a sports fan to appreciate the tremendous difference a positive attitude makes. Victory doesn't always go to the strongest or fastest but to the one who wants it most. A positive attitude means believing in miracles. In sports, there are countless stories of people who overcame overwhelming odds to achieve their personal best. These people conceived the inconceivable, and then did it. When we hear of these triumphs, our usual response is "Unbelievable!"

With the proper attitude, you can do great things. Penn State Football coach Joe Paterno describes this phenomenon: "The power of concentrating your brain, your whole body, your whole nervous system, your adrenaline, all your will on a single goal is an almost unbeatable concentration of force." David may have understood this before he went up against Goliath. After watching the 1980 United States Olympic Hockey team win the gold medal in Lake Placid, I know I do. Anything is possible.

A positive attitude means making the best of your abilities. Pete Rose was not born with great strength, size, or speed. His God-given talents were few. His most important talent was his attitude. No one got more out of himself on a baseball diamond than Pete Rose. As Pulitzer Prize winning sports columnist Jim Murray wrote, "God made Babe Ruth and Mickey Mantle baseball players. Pete Rose made Pete Rose one."

A competitor finds a way to win. Competitors take bad breaks and use them to drive themselves just that much harder. Quitters take bad breaks and use them as reasons to give up. It's all a matter of pride. You'll never know what you can do unless you try. Life is short. Try as hard as you can. You owe it to your future patients and, especially, to yourself.

A positive attitude means adopting the work ethic. The only place where success comes before hard work is in the dictionary. Athletics teaches the self-discipline of hard work and sacrifice necessary to reach a goal. Nowadays, too many people are looking for a short cut. They want a free ride, a handout. For athletes this shouldn't be true because they know what it takes. There are no short cuts to success—just the blood, sweat, and tears that produce results. Life resembles athletics: You must work hard to achieve anything. It's like the bank. Unless you make a deposit, you cannot make a withdrawal.

Some people say that good things happen to those who wait. I say that great things happen to those who work. American poet Robert Frost once wrote, "The world is full of willing people, some willing to work, others willing to let them." Boy, was he right. Don't spend your professional life on the sidelines watching others achieve greatness. Do it yourself. Make the effort to work harder to overcome your weaknesses.

A positive attitude means never becoming complacent and satisfied with the job you do. Always try to do it better. Develop an insatiable appetite for perfection. Like the writer who writes a bestseller wants to create another one, like the painter who creates a masterpiece wants to paint another one, like the lawyer who wins the most prominent case in the nation wants to try another one—it doesn't mean they have to do it. The great ones want to do it again. Great EMTs never end their search for better ways to treat their patients.

What are your weaknesses? Successful dieters say the best way to get started on a diet is to stand naked in front of a mirror (without holding in your stomach) for an honest evaluation. That's what this book is all about. Be self-critical and make small improvements in those areas that need it most. Be patient. As any weekend golfer can tell you, improvement comes slowly. The difference between the possible and the impossible lies in your determination. You must have goals and dreams if you are ever going to do anything in this world. Set your goals in life, and go after them with all the drive, self-confidence, and determination that you possess.

Good luck!

CHAPTER 1

Roles and Responsibilities of the EMT-Intermediate

QUESTIONS
1. EMS prior to the late 1960s was characterized by:
   A. fast, horizontal transport.
   B. an elaborate communications network.
   C. intensive training programs.
   D. strict medical direction.

2. How did Dr. J. Frank Pantridge of Belfast, Ireland plant the seed for prehospital emergency care?
   A. He trained the first EMT-Intermediates.
   B. He brought ALS to the patient.
   C. He developed a way to send ECG by radio.
   D. He authored the "White Paper."

3. The physician credited with training the first EMT-Intermediates in the United States is:
   A. Dr. J. Frank Pantridge.
   B. Dr. Eugene Nagel.
   C. Dr. Mickey Eisenberg.
   D. Dr. Jeffrey Clawson.

4. The rules that govern the conduct of members of a particular group or occupation are called:
   A. ethics.
   B. morals.
   C. standards.
   D. principles.

5. Professionalism is exhibited by all of the following **EXCEPT**:
   A. setting high standards.
   B. seeking self-improvement.

2 Chapter 1: Roles and Responsibilities of the EMT-Intermediate

C. earning the respect of your peers.
D. aiming for the minimum standard.

6. Which of the following is NOT an on-scene duty of the EMT-Intermediate?
   A. Patient care.
   B. Leadership.
   C. Certification.
   D. Customer service.

7. The process by which an agency or association grants recognition to an individual who has met its qualifications is known as:
   A. licensure.
   B. certification.
   C. reciprocity.
   D. censure.

8. The process by which a governmental agency grants permission to engage in a given occupation to an individual who has attained the degree of competency required to ensure the public's protection is known as:
   A. licensure.
   B. certification.
   C. reciprocity.
   D. censure.

9. The process by which an agency grants credentials to an individual who has comparable credentials from another agency is known as:
   A. licensure.
   B. certification.
   C. reciprocity.
   D. consensus.

10. NASAR, NAEMSP, and NAEMT are examples of:
    A. professional organizations.
    B. EMS journals.
    C. licensing agencies.
    D. national testing agencies.

11. Which of the following is NOT a responsibility of the National Registry?
    A. Administering testing materials.
    B. Establishing national standards.
    C. Assisting in evaluating training programs.
    D. Licensing and certifying EMT's in each state.

12. EMT-Intermediates spend the majority of their time
    A. answering emergency calls.
    B. in self-preparation.
    C. providing patient care.
    D. answering systems-abuse calls.

ANSWERS

1. ANS—A

Prior to the late 1960s, EMS was characterized by fast horizontal transport, crude rescue, and little training. There was no physician direction, communications, or specialized emergency medical knowledge. When people died, it was "meant to be." The public did not expect much prehospital care and did not receive much.

2. ANS—B *IEC—8*

Dr. J. Frank Pantridge, a cardiologist at the Royal Victoria Hospital in Belfast, Northern Ireland, introduced the concept of bringing advanced cardiac life support to the patient in the field. His paper, titled "A Mobile Intensive Care Unit," established the basis for future prehospital efforts.

3. ANS—B *IEC—8*

Dr. Eugene Nagel, of the University of Miami School of Medicine, trained a group of Miami firefighters to be the first EMT-Intermediates. He developed the first telemetry unit from an old milk crate and was the first to extend his medical license to paraprofessionals in the field. Since then, formal training programs have been organized nationwide. Today over 400 EMT-Intermediate training programs exist in the United States.

4. ANS—A *IEC—9*

Ethics are the rules of conduct that govern members of a particular group or profession. Examples of ethical codes for EMS include the EMT Code of Ethics and the EMT Oath. They are not laws, or morals, but rather guidelines for proper behavior expected from professionals.

5. ANS—D *IEC—12*

Professionalism describes the conduct or qualities that characterize a practitioner in a particular field or occupation. Professionals take pride in their work and earn the respect of their peers by the way they conduct daily business. They are the role models who set high standards for themselves and their colleagues. The professional EMT-Intermediate promotes only excellent quality patient care.

6. ANS—C *IEC—15*

On-scene duties of the EMT-Intermediate include size-up and assuring scene safety; needs determination; communication; patient assessment; assigning priorities of care; developing a treatment plan; leading the patient care team; initiating basic and advanced life support procedures; assessing the effects of treatment; establishing contact with the medical control physician; directing and coordinating patient transportation; and maintaining rapport with patients, support agencies, and hospital personnel. Maintaining current certification is an off-duty responsibility.

7. ANS—B *IEC—17*

Certification is the process by which an agency or association grants recognition to an individual who has met its qualifications. It is not a license to practice, but rather a statement that a person has fulfilled predetermined requirements. Each EMT-Intermediate must maintain current certification by following the guidelines established by the certifying agency.

8. ANS—A *IEC—17*

A license is permission to engage in a given occupation. A governmental agency grants licensure to individuals who have attained the degree of competency required to ensure the public's protection. A state grants licenses to teachers, physicians, nurses, and barbers. Some states also license their EMT-Intermediates.

9. ANS—C *IEC—17*

Reciprocity is the process by which an agency grants automatic certification or licensure to an individual who has comparable credentials from another agency.

Some states grant automatic EMT-Intermediate certification to a person who holds an EMT-Intermediate card from another state. Others grant certification to individuals who are nationally registered.

10. ANS—A *IEC—19*

Belonging to a national EMS organization is an excellent way to communicate with members from other parts of the country. Some national organizations include the National Association for Search and Rescue (NASAR), the National Association of EMS Physicians (NAEMSP), and the National Association of EMTs (NAEMT).

11. ANS—D *IEC—19*

The National Registry is an agency that prepares and administers standardized testing materials, assists in developing and evaluating training programs, establishes the qualifications for registration, and serves as a major tool for reciprocity by establishing the national minimum standard for competency.

12. ANS—B *IEC—20*

Professional EMT-Intermediates spend the vast majority of their time preparing for the next emergency call. Being an EMT-Intermediate means accepting the responsibility of being the leader in the prehospital phase of emergency medical care. Leaders understand that the key to performance is preparation. The end of the training program marks only the beginning of the EMT-Intermediate's education.

CHAPTER 2

Emergency Medical Services Systems

QUESTIONS

1. The type of EMS system in which various levels of responders are dispatched to calls depending on the severity of the situation is known as a:
   A. multi-level system.
   B. standard system.
   C. call screening system.
   D. tiered system.

2. In 1966, the "White Paper":
   A. deleted all federal funding for EMS.
   B. outlined deficiencies in emergency care.
   C. established the "15 components" of an EMS system.
   D. appropriated over $200 million for EMS.

3. Which of the following was **NOT** a necessary requirement to receive federal dollars from the EMS Systems Act of 1973?
   A. Training.
   B. Mutual aid.
   C. Consumer participation.
   D. Medical direction.

4. State EMS agencies are usually responsible for all of the following **EXCEPT**:
   A. contracting local medical directors.
   B. enacting EMS legislation.
   C. licensing and certifying field personnel.
   D. enforcing statewide EMS regulations.

5. Who has the ultimate authority in all patient care-related issues in a local EMS system?

A. State EMS Director.
B. System Medical Director.
C. Chief EMS person on-duty.
D. Local EMS Coordinator.

6. Which of the following is an example of direct medical control?
A. Developing protocols and standing orders.
B. Consulting with the physician on the radio during an emergency call.
C. Designing Continuing Quality Improvement activities.
D. Conducting chart reviews.

7. EMT-Intermediate field interventions that are completed before contacting the medical control physician are known as:
A. indirect medical control orders.
B. the 4 "Ts."
C. intervener physician protocols.
D. standing orders.

8. Which of the following are important areas in which to educate the public?
A. How to easily access the EMS system.
B. How to initiate basic life support procedures.
C. How to recognize a medical emergency.
D. All of the above.

9. Which of the following is a component of a modern E-911 system?
A. Instant call-back capabilities.
B. Automatic caller location.
C. Instant routing of the call.
D. All of the above.

10. A system of emergency medical dispatching introduced by the Salt Lake City Fire Department that standardizes every aspect of dispatching emergency vehicles is known as:
A. priority dispatching.
B. pre-arrival dispatching.
C. triage dispatching.
D. call screening.

11. System status management determines ambulance placement based on:
A. projected call volumes and locations.
B. signed contracts.
C. political sectors.
D. geographical boundaries.

12. Which of the following is a nationally recognized level of EMT?
A. EMT—Critical Care.
B. EMT—Ambulance.
C. EMT—Basic.
D. EMT—Cardiac Technician.

13. Which governmental agency develops training curricula for all EMT training programs?
A. Department of Education.
B. Department of Transportation.

C. Department of Health and Human Services.
D. Department of Public Safety.

14. In 1983, the American College of Surgeons established guidelines for:
   A. ambulance specifications.
   B. response times for trauma.
   C. BLS equipment to be carried in ambulances.
   D. the use of the pneumatic antishock garment.

15. The KKK standards deal with:
   A. ambulance safety and design.
   B. minimum standard medical protocols.
   C. training and education of field personnel.
   D. air evacuation of trauma victims.

16. In 1970, the MAST program was established to:
   A. raise the blood pressure in shock victims.
   B. bring military air medical transport capabilities to civilian accident scenes.
   C. lower the evacuation times for wounded soldiers in Vietnam.
   D. to raise funds to establish regional EMS systems.

17. Research in EMS is important in order to:
   A. justify future funding allocations.
   B. scientifically evaluate EMT-Intermediate care.
   C. weigh the benefits versus the risks of certain prehospital treatments.
   D. all of the above.

18. Hospital categorization is important because:
   A. not every patient can afford every hospital.
   B. receiving facilities have varying capabilities.
   C. not all patients can be transported to the appropriate facility.
   D. it is impossible to match patient needs with hospital resources.

19. Quality assurance differs from quality improvement in that:
   A. quality assurance deals with patient perceptions of quality.
   B. quality improvement is an objective look at clinical care.
   C. quality assurance is often viewed as punitive and negative.
   D. quality improvement does not elicit customer satisfaction information.

20. The Public Utility Model and the Failsafe Franchise are examples of:
   A. CQI programs.
   B. KKK standards.
   C. system financing.
   D. dispatching protocols.

ANSWERS

1. ANS—D   *IEC—27*

A "tiered" system is one in which basic life support first responders are dispatched unless advanced life support is needed. In that case, both are simultaneously dispatched to the emergency and the first responders initiate care until the higher level arrives.

2. ANS—B *IEC—27*

In 1966, the National Academy of Sciences—National Research Council published a paper entitled "Accidental Death and Disability, the Neglected Disease of Modern Society." The "White Paper," as it is better known, focused national attention on the problem of inadequate emergency medical care. It suggested guidelines for developing regional EMS systems, training prehospital care providers, and upgrading ambulances and their equipment. This landmark publication set off a series of federal and private funding initiatives.

3. ANS—D *IEC—28*

Of the 15 necessary components, the two that are missing are the most interesting. The authors of this legislation never foresaw the need to ensure medical direction and physician involvement in EMS system design. Neither did they see the need to ensure the financial stability of these programs in the event that the "soft" federal dollars became scarce. Both of these oversights led EMS in the wrong direction.

4. ANS—A *IEC—29*

State EMS agencies are typically responsible for allocating funding to local systems, acting legislation concerning the prehospital practice of medicine, licensing and certifying field providers, enforcing all state EMS regulations, and appointing regional advisory councils. Hiring a local system medical director is the responsibility of the local EMS administrative agency.

5. ANS—B *IEC—30*

The local EMS system medical director is the ultimate authority in all patient care-related issues in the local EMS system. All prehospital patient care activities are extensions of this physician's license. Only a physician is licensed to practice medicine. This doctrine is known as "delegation of authority."

6. ANS—B *IEC—30*

Direct medical control exists when prehospital providers communicate directly with the physician at a medical control or resource hospital. The physician's direction is usually based on established protocols from managing specific problems. This physician assumes responsibility and gives treatment orders for patients. Direct medical control physicians should be experienced in emergency medicine.

7. ANS—D *IEC—32*

EMT-Intermediate field interventions that are completed before contacting the medical control physician are known as standing orders. Standing orders are established by indirect medical control prior to the emergency call. These allow EMT-Intermediates to perform certain procedures without a direct order from the base station physician.

8. ANS—D *IEC—33*

The public is an essential but often overlooked component of an EMS system. An EMS system should have a plan for educating the public about recognizing an emergency situation, accessing the EMS system, and initiating basic life support procedures.

9. ANS—D *IEC—34*

The basic emergency telephone number, 911, is a toll-free telephone service that enables the caller to dial three digits to reach a single public safety answering point. Enhanced 911 gives automatic location of the caller, instant routing of the call to the appropriate emergency service agency, and instant call back capabilities if the caller hangs up too soon.

10. ANS—A *IEC—38*

A system of emergency medical dispatching introduced by the Salt Lake City Fire Department that standardizes every aspect of dispatching emergency vehicles is known as "priority dispatching." In this system, medical dispatchers are trained to medically interrogate the distressed caller, prioritize symptoms, select the appropriate response, and give life-saving pre-arrival instructions. These protocols are designed and approved by the system medical director.

11. ANS—A *IEC—38*

System status management is an emergency medical dispatching tool used to place ambulances and crews strategically around an EMS coverage area. The system status manager relies on projected call volumes and locations rather than on geographical or political traditions. It is used to reduce response times.

12. ANS—C *IEC—39*

The National Registry of EMTs recognizes and the Department of Transportation develops training curricula for three levels of field providers: EMT-Basic, EMT-Intermediate, and EMT-Paramedic. There exist, however, approximately 30 various levels of field providers nationwide.

13. ANS—B *IEC—39*

Training curricula for EMT training programs are developed by the United States Department of Transportation. In 1966, Congress passed the National Highway Safety Act, which forced the states to develop regional EMS systems or risk losing federal highway construction funds. The Department of Transportation was entrusted with developing the training curricula for these programs.

14. ANS—C *IEC—41*

In 1983, the American College of Surgeons Committee on Trauma recommended a standard set of equipment to be carried by providers of basic life support services. In 1988, the American College of Emergency Physicians published a recommended list of advanced life support supplies and equipment to be carried on ALS units. Both sets of recommendations serve as excellent guidelines for any prehospital EMS system.

15. ANS—A *IEC—41*

In 1974, responding to a request from the Department of Transportation, the General Services Administration developed the KKK standards, which established federal specifications for ambulances. The original guidelines and the subsequent revisions were aimed at improving ambulance design and safety features.

16. ANS—B *IEC—43*

In 1970, the Military Assistance to Safety and Traffic (MAST) program was established. This demonstration project set up 35 programs nationwide to test the feasibility of using military helicopters and paramedical personnel in civilian medical emergencies.

17. ANS—D *IEC—46*

In order to provide a scientific basis for prehospital EMS, a formal ongoing research program is an essential component of the system. Research is necessary to justify future funding allocations, to scientifically evaluate EMT-Intermediate care, and to weigh the benefits versus the risks of certain prehospital treatments.

18. ANS—B *IEC—47*

Since all hospitals are not all equal in emergency and support service capabilities, hospital categorization is an important component of an EMS system. It identifies the readiness and capability of a hospital and its staff to receive and effectively treat emergency patients. Categorization originated from the realization that patients have varying degrees of illness and injury and that receiving facilities have varying capabilities to provide initial or definitive care.

19. ANS—C *IEC—45*

Quality assurance programs are primarily designed to maintain continuous monitoring and measurement of the quality of clinical care delivered. They emphasize evaluation of response times, adherence to protocols, patient survival, and other indicators. They are often viewed as punitive and negative.

20. ANS—C *IEC—50*

The public utility model and the fail safe franchise are examples of system financing. In these systems municipalities establish the design and standards for the contract bid and periodically, usually every three or four years, hold wholesale competition for the market.

CHAPTER 3

Medical Legal Considerations in Emergency Care

QUESTIONS

1. Homicide and rape are examples of wrongs against society and would be tried in:
   A. criminal court.
   B. tort court.
   C. civil court.
   D. none of the above.

2. Which of the following would be an example of a tort case?
   A. Divorce.
   B. Suicide.
   C. Contract dispute.
   D. Malpractice.

3. EMT-Intermediates could find themselves involved in which types of legal cases?
   A. Tort cases.
   B. Civil cases.
   C. Criminal cases.
   D. All of the above.

4. A "Medical Practice Act":
   A. defines the scope of practice for allied health care professionals.
   B. is a national standard for allied health care professionals.
   C. outlines ethical behavior guidelines for medical paraprofessionals.
   D. is unecessary in states that license their EMT-Intermediates.

5. The doctrine of "delegation of authority" states that:
   A. EMT-Intermediates may practice independently.
   B. EMT-Intermediates may only practice under the license of a physician.

C. EMT-Intermediates cannot be found criminally liable for practicing without a license.
D. EMT-Intermediates do not require a "Medical Practice Act."

6. Laws that protect health care workers from liability in the event they stop and render roadside care are known as:
   A. Good Samaritan laws.
   B. *Res ipsa loquitor* laws.
   C. Delegation of Authority laws.
   D. Negligence laws.

7. If a question arises concerning the validity of "Do Not Resuscitate" orders or "Living Wills," the EMT-Intermediate should:
   A. contact medical control.
   B. ignore all such orders and run the code.
   C. accept and honor all such orders.
   D. run a "slow code" in these cases.

8. Negligence is defined as:
   A. lawsuits involving no physical harm.
   B. deviating from the standard of care.
   C. failing to prove proximate cause.
   D. all of the above.

9. Which of the following is NOT a necessary component of a successful negligence suit?
   A. Duty to act.
   B. Breach of duty.
   C. Proximate cause.
   D. Unlawful consent.

10. In *res ipsa loquitor*, the burden of proof rests with the:
    A. plaintiff.
    B. defendant.
    C. medical advisory council.
    D. district attorney.

11. Informed consent means:
    A. the adult patient is mentally competent.
    B. the patient understands the treatment and the risks.
    C. the patient agrees to the treatment.
    D. all of the above.

12. Which of the following would NOT fall under the concept of implied consent?
    A. An unconscious diabetic in insulin shock.
    B. A 5-year-old in anaphylactic shock with no parent present.
    C. A mentally retarded person with bilateral fractured femurs.
    D. A diabetic who awakens following 50% Dextrose therapy and refuses transport.

13. Failure to formally transfer the patient to medical staff in the emergency department could place the EMT-Intermediate in danger of being sued for:
    A. false imprisonment.

B. unlawful consent.
C. abandonment.
D. patient endangerment.

14. Threatening to defibrillate a patient if he does not quiet down could place an EMT-Intermediate in danger of being sued for:
A. assault.
B. battery.
C. libel.
D. slander.

15. Starting an IV on a competent patient who absolutely refuses one could place the EMT-Intermediate in danger of being sued for:
A. assault.
B. battery.
C. libel.
D. slander.

16. Transporting a patient to the hospital against his will could place the EMT-Intermediate in danger of being sued for:
A. false imprisonment.
B. kidnapping.
C. unlawful consent.
D. assault and battery.

17. Stating on the air that "We've got Frank Jones again, and he's drunk and obnoxious as usual" could place the EMT-Intermediate in danger of being sued for:
A. assault.
B. battery.
C. libel.
D. slander.

18. Writing on the run sheet that a certain patient "probably has AIDS from deviant homosexual activity" could place the EMT-Intermediate in danger of being sued for:
A. assault.
B. defamation of character.
C. libel.
D. slander.

19. Which of the following statements is true concerning prehospital documentation?
A. If you don't write it down, you did not do it.
B. A well-documented run sheet can be your best defense in court.
C. Intentional alterations of the run sheet are considered admissions of guilt.
D. All of the above.

20. An EMT-Intermediate's best defense against potential legal liability is:
A. purchasing medical malpractice insurance.
B. documenting as little as possible on the run sheet.
C. relying on Good Samaritan immunity.
D. practicing excellent quality prehospital care.

ANSWERS

1. ANS—A *IEC—54*

Criminal law deals with crimes against society and their punishments. Criminal litigations are legal actions taken by the state against the offending individual. Homicide and rape are examples of criminal wrongs. To convict requires proof beyond a reasonable doubt.

2. ANS—D *IEC—55*

Tort law, a branch of civil law, deals with civil wrongs committed by one individual against another. A medical malpractice suit is an example of tort against an EMT-Intermediate. Unlike a criminal case, only a preponderance of evidence (50% +1) is needed to win the case.

3. ANS—D *IEC—55*

EMT-Intermediates may become involved in any aspect of the legal system. They may be called as witnesses in a criminal offense, asked to testify in a civil matter, or named in malpractice litigation.

4. ANS—A *IEC—56*

A "Medical Practice Act" is specific state legislation that defines the scope and role of the EMT-Intermediate and other allied health care professionals. It establishes the requirements for those who will be allowed to practice and identifies certification and licensing procedures. Medical Practice acts differ from state to state.

5. ANS—B *IEC—56*

EMT-Intermediates are not licensed to practice independently. They may only function under the supervision of a licensed physician through delegation of authority. This supervision may be direct (in person, on radio) or indirect (protocols, standing orders). Failure to adhere to this requirement could make the EMT-Intermediate criminally liable for practicing medicine without a license. In some states, this constitutes a felony, punishable by fines or imprisonment.

6. ANS—A *IEC—56*

Laws that protect off-duty health care workers from liability in the event they stop and render roadside care are known as "Good Samaritan Laws." A person is immune from liability for assisting at the scene of a medical emergency if he or she acts in good faith, is not grossly negligent, and does not accept payment for services. Unfortunately, gross negligence is a subjective term and the plaintiff's attorney will portray the EMT-Intermediate as such. A jury of non-medical civilians will listen to testimony and decide the outcome. In many cases, the Good Samaritan defense has not held up in court.

7. ANS—A *IEC—58*

When questions concerning the validity of "Do Not Resuscitate" orders or "Living Wills" arise in the field, EMT-Intermediates should contact medical control. EMT-Intermediates don't have the legal authority and are not in the position to evaluate the validity of such documents.

8. ANS—B *IEC—60*

Negligence is defined as deviating from accepted standards of care. In medicine, negligence is synonymous with malpractice. EMT-Intermediates can be negligent by not performing to the standard of care (failing to immobilize the c-spine); by performing beyond their training and certification (any skill not approved by the local medical director), or by substandard performance (unrecognized esophageal intubation of a breathing patient).

Chapter 3: Medical Legal Considerations in Emergency Care **15**

9. ANS—D *IEC—60*

To win a negligence case the plaintiff's attorney must prove that an EMT-Intermediate's breach of duty caused harm to the patient. Once again, in a tort case, only a preponderance of evidence is needed to win.

10. ANS—B *IEC—61*

When the doctrine of *res ipsa loquitor* is invoked, the burden of proof shifts from the plaintiff to the defendant. *Res ipsa loquitor* is Latin for "The thing speaks for itself" and states that the damages could not have occurred in the absence of the EMT-Intermediate's negligence. For example, only the EMT-Intermediate could have placed the endotracheal tube into the esophagus.

11. ANS—D *IEC—61*

Informed consent must be obtained from every conscious, mentally competent adult person before treatment can be started. Informed consent means that the adult patient is mentally competent, understands the treatment and the risks, and agrees to be treated.

12. ANS—D *IEC—62*

Unconscious patients cannot express consent. When treating the unconscious patient the treatment is considered to be implied. With implied consent it is assumed that the patient would want life-saving treatment if he or she were able to provide expressed consent.

13. ANS—C *IEC—64*

Abandonment is the termination of the EMT-Intermediate-patient relationship without ensuring a mechanism for the continuation of the care. EMT-Intermediates should not initiate care and then arbitrarily discontinue it. Physically leaving a patient unattended on an emergency department stretcher may be grounds for abandonment if the patient's condition deteriorates.

14. ANS—A *IEC—64*

Assault is defined as unlawfully placing a person in apprehension of immediate bodily harm without his or her consent. Threatening to defibrillate a patient if he does not quiet down could place an EMT-Intermediate in danger of being sued for assault. Assault can be either a criminal or a civil offense.

15. ANS—B *IEC—64*

Battery is the unlawful touching of another individual without his or her consent. Starting an IV on a competent patient who absolutely refuses one could place the EMT-Intermediate in danger of being sued for battery. Battery could also be a criminal or a civil offense.

16. ANS—A *IEC—64*

Everyone has the right to be left alone. False imprisonment is defined as unlawful and unjustifiable detention. Transporting a patient to the hospital against his will could constitute false imprisonment. In these cases, EMT-Intermediates should ensure that the transportation is medically justified.

17. ANS—D *IEC—65*

Slander is the act of injuring a person's character, name, or reputation by false or malicious spoken words. Information transmitted over the radio should be limited to essential matters of patient care. The medical report should never contain the patient's name or the EMT-Intermediate's subjective opinions.

18. ANS—C *IEC—65*

Libel is the act of injuring a person's character, name, or reputation by false or malicious writings. Allegations of libel can be avoided by respecting the patient's confidentiality. The medical record should be accurate and confidential; slang and labels should be avoided. Never write anything on the run report that might be construed as libel.

19. ANS—D *IEC—66*

A complete, well-written run report is an EMT-Intermediate's best protection in a malpractice proceeding. To the court, observations and treatments not documented on the run report were not performed. The medical records should never be altered, as it amounts to an admission of guilt by the EMT-Intermediate.

20. ANS—D *IEC—66*

An EMT-Intermediate's best defense against potential legal liability is practicing the highest quality of patient care, which includes good documentation.

CHAPTER 4

Medical Terminology

QUESTIONS Give the plain English meaning for the following medical terms:

1. Adenopathy _____
2. Neuralgia _____
3. Angioplasty _____
4. Arthritis _____
5. Myasthenia _____
6. Bronchitis _____
7. Bursitis _____
8. Myocardial _____
9. Pericardiocentesis _____
10. Costochondritis _____
11. Intradermal _____
12. Abduction _____
13. Gastroenterology _____
14. Erythrocyte _____
15. Anesthesia _____
16. Afebrile _____
17. Hematuria _____
18. Hydrocephalic _____
19. Hysterectomy _____
20. Idioventricular _____

21. Nephrology
22. Intraosseous
23. Polyphagia
24. Pneuonectomy
25. Rhinorrhea
26. Arteriosclerosis
27. Hemostasis
28. Tachypnea
29. Adduction
30. Antihistamine
31. Bilateral
32. Bradycardia
33. Cerebrospinal
34. Contralateral
35. Dyspnea
36. Endocardium
37. Epidermis
38. Eupnea
39. Extrasystole
40. Hematoma
41. Hemiplegia
42. Hypoglycemia
43. Intravascular
44. Isotonic
45. Leukocyte
46. Oliguria
47. Periorbital
48. Arthroscopy
49. Retroperitoneum
50. Vasopressor
51. Sublingual
52. Supraclavicular
53. Transtracheal
54. Unilateral
55. Tracheostomy
56. Laryngoscopy
57. Psychosis
58. Aphasia
59. Photophobic
60. Dysrhythmia

61. Hypertrophy _____
62. Polyuria _____
63. Pylonephritis _____
64. Postpartum _____
65. Rhinoplasty _____

Write the common abbreviations for the following terms:

66. Before _____
67. Atherosclerotic heart disease _____
68. Against medical advice _____
69. Blood sugar _____
70. Body surface area _____
71. Bag-valve-mask _____
72. With _____
73. Cubic centimeter _____
74. Chief complaint _____
75. Centimeter _____
76. Congestive heart failure _____
77. Complains of _____
78. Carbon monoxide _____
79. Carbon dioxide _____
80. Chronic obstructive pulmonary disease _____
81. Chest pain _____
82. Cerebrospinal fluid _____
83. Carotid sinus massage _____
84. Cerebrovascular accident _____
85. Discontinue _____
86. Dyspnea on exertion _____
87. Deep vein thrombosis _____
88. Estimated date of confinement _____
89. Alcohol (ethanol) _____
90. Fracture _____
91. Gastrointestinal _____
92. Gunshot wound _____
93. Hour _____
94. Headache _____
95. History _____
96. Intramuscular _____
97. Intraosseous _____
98. Jugular venous distension _____

Chapter 4: Medical Terminology

99. Potassium _____
100. Kilogram _____
101. Keep vein open _____
102. Laceration _____
103. Lactated Ringer's _____
104. Moves all extremities well _____
105. Microgram _____
106. Milliequivalent _____
107. Milligram _____
108. Milliliter _____
109. Morphine sulfate _____
110. Sodium _____
111. Sodium chloride _____
112. No known allergies _____
113. Nitroglycerine _____
114. Nausea/vomiting _____
115. Organic brain syndrome _____
116. After _____
117. Hydrogen ion concentration _____
118. Pelvic inflammatory disease _____
119. As needed _____
120. Patient _____
121. Every _____
122. Rule out _____
123. Range of motion _____
124. Without _____
125. Signs/symptoms _____
126. Subcutaneous _____
127. Sublingual _____
128. Within normal limits _____
129. Change _____
130. Year old _____

Translate the following medical report into everyday English:

Pt. is a 45 y.o. male, AO x 4, c/o sudden onset CP and SOB x 2h. Pt. also c/o DOE, N/V, and weakness. Pt. has Hx of ASHD and AMI x2 with CHF, and TIA x 1. He takes NTG 0.4mg. SL PRN for CP. NKA. VS as follows: BP 170/80, pulse 80, respirations 28, BS clear bilaterally, skin WNL. ECG shows NSR with PVC's, BS is 120. R/O AMI. Plan - O_2 - 10 LPM, NTG 0.4 mg. SL q5 minutes PRN, MS 2 mg IV repeat PRN.

ANSWERS

1. Disease of the glands
2. Pain along a nerve
3. Blood vessel repair
4. Inflammation of a joint
5. Muscle weakness
6. Inflammation of the bronchioles
7. Inflammation of the bursa
8. Pertaining to the heart muscle
9. Puncturing and draining the pericardium
10. Inflammation of the rib cartilage
11. Within the layers of the skin
12. Movement away from the body
13. The study of the GI tract
14. Red blood cell
15. Without feeling
16. Without fever
17. Blood in the urine
18. Excess water in the brain
19. Surgical removal of the uterus
20. Originating in the ventricles
21. The study of the kidneys
22. Within the bone
23. Excessive eating
24. Surgical removal of a lung
25. Runny nose
26. Hardening of the arteries
27. Standing blood
28. Rapid breathing
29. Movement toward the body
30. Against histamine (blocker)
31. On both sides
32. Slow heart (rate)
33. The brain and spine
34. On the opposite side
35. Difficulty in breathing

36. The inner heart (lining)
37. The outer skin (layer)
38. Normal breathing
39. Extra contraction (beat)
40. A blood tumor (pocket)
41. One-sided paralysis
42. Low blood sugar
43. Within a blood vessel
44. The same tone (concentration)
45. White blood cell
46. Little urine (production)
47. Around the eye orbit
48. Looking into a joint
49. Behind the peritoneum
50. An agent that constricts a blood vessel
51. Under the tongue
52. Above the clavicles
53. Across the trachea
54. On one side
55. A surgical opening into the trachea
56. Looking into the larynx
57. A mental disorder
58. Inability to speak
59. Fear of light
60. Disorganized rhythm (cardiac)
61. Overnourishment (enlargement)
62. Frequent urination
63. Kidney infection
64. After birth bleeding
65. Repair of the nose (plastic surgery)
66. ā
67. ASHD
68. AMA
69. BS
70. BSA
71. BVM

72. c̄
73. cc
74. CC
75. CM
76. CHF
77. c/o
78. CO
79. CO_2
80. COPD
81. CP
82. CSF
83. CSM
84. CVA
85. D/C
86. DOE
87. DVT
88. EDC
89. ETOH
90. Fx
91. GI
92. GSW
93. h
94. H/A
95. Hx
96. IM
97. IO
98. JVD
99. K^+
100. Kg
101. KVO
102. LAC
103. LR
104. MOEW
105. Mcg
106. mEq
107. Mg

108. MI

109. MS

110. Na⁺

111. NaCl

112. NKA

113. NTG

114. N/V

115. OBS

116. p̄

117. pH

118. PID

119. PRN

120. Pt

121. q̄

122. R/O

123. ROM

124. s̄

125. S/S

126. SC

127. SL

128. WNL

129. D

130. y.o.

The patient is a 45-year-old male, alert and oriented to person, place, and time, who complains of a sudden onset of chest pain and shortness of breath that began two hours ago. The patient also complains of dyspnea upon exertion, nausea, vomiting, and weakness. The patient has a history of atherosclerotic heart disease and has had two heart attacks with congestive heart failure, and one transient ischemic attack. He takes nitroglycerine 0.4 milligrams sublingually as needed for chest pain. He has no known allergies. His vital signs are as follows: Blood pressure 170/80, pulse 80, respirations 28, breath sounds clear bilaterally, skin within normal limits. His electrocardiogram shows normal sinus rhythm with premature ventricular contractions. Blood sugar is 120. Rule out acute myocardial infarction. Plan—oxygen at 10 liters per minute; nitroglycerine 0.4 milligrams sublingually every 5 minutes as needed; Morphine sulfate 2 milligrams intravenously; repeat as needed.

CHAPTER 5

EMS Communications

QUESTIONS

1. The principle transmitter and receiver of a communications system is known as the:
   A. mobile radio.
   B. base station.
   C. satellite.
   D. repeater.

2. Which of the following will **NOT** impede the range of radio transmissions?
   A. Flatlands.
   B. Mountains.
   C. High buildings.
   D. Dense foliage.

3. A device that receives a transmission from a low-power source on one frequency and retransmits it at a higher power on another frequency is a/an:
   A. mobile transmitter.
   B. repeater.
   C. encoder.
   D. decoder.

4. The process by which low power transmissions are selected by the receiver that picks up the strongest signal and boosts the signal to the base station is known as:
   A. decoding.
   B. boosting.
   C. encoding.
   D. voting.

5. A device that transmits specific tones to activate certain radios is called a/an:
   A. encoder.
   B. voter.
   C. repeater.
   D. decoder.
6. A radio pager is an example of a/an:
   A. encoder.
   B. decoder.
   C. repeater.
   D. voter.
7. Which of the following is an advantage of using cellular communications?
   A. 12 lead ECGs can be transmitted.
   B. FAX and computer messages can be transmitted.
   C. Dedicated EMT-Intermediate lines can be established.
   D. All of the above.
8. A group of radio frequencies close together is called a:
   A. band.
   B. spectrum.
   C. multiplex.
   D. UHF configuration.
9. Which of the following is not an EMS frequency range?
   A. VHF-Lo.
   B. VHF-High.
   C. UHF.
   D. AM.
10. Which of the following radio frequency ranges offers the clearest communications with the least interference?
    A. 30–50 MHz.
    B. 150–170 MHz.
    C. 450–470 MHz.
    D. 800+ MHz.
11. Trunking is a communications term that describes:
    A. computerized frequency allocation.
    B. hard-wiring for ambulance radios.
    C. base station radio procedures.
    D. multiple antennae installation.
12. Which of the "med channels" are designated for field-to-physician communications?
    A. 1–8.
    B. 9–10.
    C. All 10.
    D. 1–2.
13. Transmitting the patient's ECG over the air is a process known as:
    A. demodulation.
    B. voting.
    C. biotelemetry.
    D. trunking.

14. A modulator:
  A. converts radio tones into ECG voltage changes.
  B. converts ECG voltage changes into radio tones.
  C. is found in the hospital base station.
  D. displays its signal on an oscilloscope.

15. Which of the following can cause ECG interference?
  A. Loose electrodes.
  B. Muscle tremors.
  C. 60 Hz.
  D. All of the above.

16. Which of the following is true concerning radio equipment maintenance?
  A. Regular maintenance can improve the radio's life expectancy.
  B. Cleaning solvents can be used on the outer case safely.
  C. Any EMT-Intermediate can perform simple repairs on the radio.
  D. Simply dropping a radio rarely causes damage.

17. The governmental agency that regulates all radio communications is the:
  A. Department of Transportation.
  B. Department of Communications.
  C. Federal Communications Commission.
  D. National Association of Broadcasting.

ANSWERS

1. ANS—B *IEC—97*

The principle transmitter and receiver of a communications system is known as the base station. It is usually the most powerful radio in the system with output typically 45–275 watts. Some base stations are multiple channel systems but most can only communicate on one channel at a time.

2. ANS—A *IEC—97*

Transmissions over flatland or water will not impede the range. Transmissions over mountains, through dense foliage, or in urban areas of large buildings will decrease the range.

3. ANS—B *IEC—99*

A repeater is a device that receives a transmission from a low power portable or a mobile radio on one frequency and re-transmits it at a higher power on another frequency. Repeaters are important in large geographical areas because portable and mobile radios may not have enough range to communicate with each other, with medical control, or with the dispatcher.

4. ANS—D *IEC—100*

Many large EMS systems have more than one repeater. Often, when a mobile unit transmits, more than one repeater will pick up the transmission. A system designed so that the repeater receiving the strongest signal will transmit the message is known as voting.

5. ANS—A *IEC—101*

A device for generating unique codes or tones that are recognized by another radio's decoder is called an encoder. An encoder is similar to a telephone keypad. When activated by pressing the buttons, it sends specific tones over the air.

6. ANS—B *IEC—101*

A device that receives and recognizes unique codes or tones sent over the air is called a decoder. Only the sequence of tones specific for that decoder will activate it. Most radio pagers work on this principle.

7. ANS—D *IEC—101*

Many EMS systems are using cellular communications. Advantages include: the ability to transmit 12 lead EKGs, fax, and computer messages, and the ability to establish dedicated EMT-Intermediate lines into the base station hospital.

8. ANS—A *IEC—103*

A group of radio frequencies close together on the electromagnetic spectrum is called a band. Some examples of radio bands are AM, FM, citizen band, short wave, UHF, and VHF.

9. ANS—D *IEC—103*

The FCC has designated certain bands for use in EMS. They include VHF low, 30–50 MHz; VHF high, 150–170 MHz; UHF 450–470 MHz; and a new band in the 800 MHz range.

10. ANS—D *IEC—102*

As a rule, the lower the band the farther the range, but the more interference. The clearest communications in EMS can be utilized in the 800 megahertz range UHF. UHF transmissions have less range than VHF, but they are less susceptable to interference.

11. ANS—A *IEC—103*

In a trunked system, all frequencies are pooled together. A computer routes a radio transmission to the first available frequency. All subsequent transmissions are routed in the same manner. This eliminates the need to search for unused frequencies.

12. ANS—A *IEC—104*

The FCC has designated EMS channels for use nationwide on the UHF band. Channels 1–8 are designated for field-to-physician communications. Channels 9–10 are for dispatching purposes.

TABLE 5-1	DESIGNATED EMS CHANNELS		
Channel	Transmit Frequency	Receive Frequency	Usage
MED 1	463.000 MHz	468.000 MHz	EMT/MD
MED 2	463.025 MHz	468.025 MHz	EMT/MD
MED 3	463.050 MHz	468.050 MHz	EMT/MD
MED 4	463.075 MHz	468.075 MHz	EMT/MD
MED 5	463.100 MHz	468.100 MHz	EMT/MD
MED 6	463.125 MHz	468.125 MHz	EMT/MD
MED 7	463.150 MHz	468.150 MHz	EMT/MD
MED 8	463.175 MHz	468.175 MHz	EMT/MD
MED 9	462.950 MHz	467.950 MHz	DISPATCH
MED 10	462.975 MHz	467.975 MHz	DISPATCH

13. ANS—C *IEC—103*

The process of transmitting physiological data such as an ECG over distance, usually by radio, is known as biotelemetry. An example of this is the EMT-Intermediate transmitting the ECG over the air to the base station physician in the hospital.

14. ANS—B *IEC—104*

A device that transforms electrical energy into sound waves is known as a modulator. The patient's biotelemetry radio is an example of a modulator. It transforms the patient's ECG voltage changes into radio tones, which are then transmitted to the hospital.

15. ANS—D *IEC—104*

Biotelemetry communications are subject to interference by such things as muscle tremors, loose electrodes, 60 hertz interference, fluctuations in transmitter power, and by the transmission of voice communications while telemetry is in progress.

16. ANS—A *IEC—104*

Radio equipment is expensive and fragile. A regular schedule of maintenance and cleaning will improve its appearance and life expectancy. Careful handling can increase its longevity and improve its performance.

17. ANS—C *IEC—105*

The Federal Communications Commission is the governmental agency responsible for assigning frequencies, regulating all radios, and controlling all radio communications in the United States.

CHAPTER 6

General Patient Assessment and Initial Management

QUESTIONS

1. Paradoxical chest wall movement would indicate:
   A. flail chest.
   B. hemothorax.
   C. pneumothorax.
   D. traumatic asphyxia.

2. In the healthy adult at rest, normal respiration should occur at a rate of _____ per minute.
   A. 16–22.
   B. 12–20.
   C. 24.
   D. 60–100.

3. The healthy adult at rest breathes in approximately _____ ml of air.
   A. 500
   B. 150
   C. 800
   D. 350

4. Exaggerated abdominal movement during breathing may indicate:
   A. spinal cord injury.
   B. diaphragmatic breathing.
   C. intercostal muscle paralysis.
   D. all of the above.

5. The presence of supraclavicular retractions suggests:
   A. hypovolemic shock.
   B. decreased blood volume.
   C. a partial airway obstruction.
   D. cardiac arrhythmias.

6. The most common cause of snoring is upper airway obstruction from:
   A. foreign bodies.
   B. stomach contents.
   C. the tongue.
   D. a swollen epiglottis.

7. Snoring is best corrected by:
   A. vigorous suctioning.
   B. repositioning the head.
   C. pumping the stomach.
   D. endotracheal intubation.

8. High-pitched "crowing" sounds caused by obstruction of the upper airway are called:
   A. wheezes.
   B. snoring.
   C. rales.
   D. stridor.

9. The whistling sounds indicative of lower airway constriction are called:
   A. wheezes.
   B. snoring.
   C. rales.
   D. stridor.

10. Your patient presents unconscious, without a gag reflex, and moving less than 6 liters/minute of air. You should do all of the following EXCEPT:
    A. Intubate the patient.
    B. Perform bag-valve-mask ventilations.
    C. Administer 100% oxygen.
    D. Complete the primary survey before treating.

11. Your patient presents with warm, pink skin, radial pulse rate of 80/minute, and capillary refill time of :02 seconds. From this information what can you conclude about her circulatory condition?
    A. It is normal.
    B. It shows signs of early circulatory compromise.
    C. It shows signs of severe circulatory collapse.
    D. None of the above.

12. Which of the following is NOT a physical exam technique?
    A. Palpation.
    B. Auscultation.
    C. Percussion.
    D. Inspection.

13. Heart sounds can best be heard by placing the stethoscope over the:
    A. apex of the heart.
    B. fourth intercostal space, right mid-clavicular line.
    C. third intercostal space, just left of the sternum.
    D. fifth intercostal space, mid-axillary line.

14. A hollow and vibrating resonance heard when percussing the chest indicates the presence of:
    A. air

B. blood.
C. pleural fluid.
D. water.

15. A black-and-bluish discoloration over the mastoid process is called:
  A. periorbital ecchymosis.
  B. Battle's sign.
  C. raccoon's eyes.
  D. Cushing's reflex.

16. A positive halo test indicates the presence of:
  A. sugar.
  B. blood.
  C. stomach contents.
  D. cerebrospinal fluid.

17. Pinpoint pupils indicate:
  A. severe brain injury.
  B. hypoxia.
  C. intracranial pressure.
  D. opiate overdose.

18. Failure of the eyes to rotate simultaneously in the same direction is called:
  A. anisocoria.
  B. dysconjugate gaze.
  C. doll's eye reflex.
  D. Battle's sign.

Match the following oral cavity fluids with their possible pathologies:

19. _____ Coffee grounds   **A.** Congestive heart failure
20. _____ Fresh blood   **B.** Respiratory infection
21. _____ Pink-tinged sputum   **C.** Bleeding in the stomach
22. _____ Green or yellow phlegm **D.** Brainstem problem
23. _____ Vomit   **E.** Upper GI hemorrhage

24. Significant jugular venous distension is evaluated with the patient's body at a _____ angle.
  A. 90°
  B. 45°
  C. 0°
  D. 180°

25. Significant JVD is indicative of
  A. hypovolemia.
  B. hypotension.
  C. cardiac tamponade.
  D. left heart failure.

26. Your patient is lying supine and his neck veins are flat. You conclude that he:
  A. has a tension pneumothorax.
  B. has right heart failure.

C. is hypovolemic.
D. has corpulmonale.

27. The presence of air just underneath the surface of the skin is known as:
   A. pulmonary emphysema.
   B. subcutaneous emphysema.
   C. crepital emphysema.
   D. ipsilateral emphysema.

28. A rapid, deep respiratory pattern may be indicative of:
   A. a head injury.
   B. extreme exertion.
   C. a diabetic problem.
   D. all of the above.

29. A series of increasing, then decreasing, breaths with periods of apnea in between is known as:
   A. Biot's.
   B. Kussmaul's.
   C. Central neurogenic hyperventilation.
   D. Cheyne-Stokes.

30. A bluish discoloration around the umbilicus is known as:
   A. Grey-Turner's sign.
   B. Cullen's sign.
   C. Cushing's reflex.
   D. Battle's sign.

31. Rebound tenderness is indicative of:
   A. peritoneal inflammation.
   B. impending aortic aneurysm rupture.
   C. solid organ inflammation.
   D. none of the above.

32. Ascites is caused by:
   A. increased portal circulation.
   B. right heart failure.
   C. cirrhosis of the liver.
   D. all of the above.

33. Presacral edema is indicative of:
   A. congestive heart failure.
   B. peritoneal irritation.
   C. cirrhosis of the liver.
   D. ruptured ipsilateral kidney.

34. Priapism is caused by:
   A. unopposed parasympathetic stimulation.
   B. spinal cord interruption.
   C. brain dysfunction.
   D. all of the above.

35. Clubbing is caused by:
   A. a chronic hypoxic condition.
   B. cardiovascular and pulmonary disease.

C. central cyanosis.
D. all of the above.

36. The difference between systolic and diastolic blood pressures is known as:
A. pulsus paradoxus.
B. mean arterial pressure.
C. central venous pressure.
D. pulse pressure.

37. If your supine patient's pulse rate rises more than 15 beats per minute when you sit him up, what should you suspect?
A. Congestive heart failure.
B. Significant blood loss.
C. Severe hypertension.
D. Coronary artery disease.

38. Patients with effective respiration should measure an oxygen saturation of:
A. 80–100 mg/kg.
B. 120 d/L.
C. 90–100 torr.
D. 96–100%.

39. In which of the following situations might your oximetry reading be misleading?
A. Severe hypothermia.
B. Carbon monoxide poisoning.
C. Hypovolemia.
D. All of the above.

40. The primary sign or symptom noticed by the patient is called the:
A. primary problem.
B. associated symptom.
C. chief complaint.
D. history of present illness.

41. When recording your patient's symptoms, it is best to use:
A. medical terminology.
B. the patient's own words.
C. your interpretation.
D. none of the above.

42. Often the pain of myocardial infarction is felt in the neck and jaw. This is known as _____ pain.
A. aggravating
B. alleviating
C. radiating
D. referred

43. The "P" in the mnemonic "AMPLE" stands for:
A. palleative factors.
B. provocative factors.
C. past medical history.
D. personal physician.

44. The "M" in the mnemonic "AMPLE" stands for:
   A. medications.
   B. medical history.
   C. monitor.
   D. movement.

45. The "A" in the mnemonic "AMPLE" stands for:
   A. allergies.
   B. attacks.
   C. aggravating factors.
   D. alleviating factors.

ANSWERS

1. ANS—A *IEC—171*

Paradoxical movement of the chest wall is when the chest wall moves in a fashion opposite to that expected. It's often seen in flail chest injuries where the flail segment moves in an opposite direction compared to the rest of the chest. This is caused by changes in pressures within the chest wall.

2. ANS—B *IEC—172*

In the healthy adult at rest normal respirations should occur at a rate of 12-20 breaths per minute.

3. ANS—A *IEC—172*

A healthy adult at rest breathes in approximately 500 ml of air. This is known as tidal volume.

4. ANS—D *IEC—172*

Exaggerated abdominal movement during breathing may indicate that the diaphragm is the only muscle being used. It may be a result of spinal cord injury or intercostal muscle paralysis in which the other muscles of breathing are no longer functional.

5. ANS—C *IEC—172*

Retraction means the act of drawing back or inward. In the case of partial airway obstruction an increased inspiratory effort causes great pressures within the chest wall. These pressures cause the tissue between the ribs and sternal notch to retract or move inward.

6. ANS—C *IEC—172*

The most common cause of snoring is upper airway obstruction from the tongue. This is generally caused by gravity moving the relaxed tongue into the posterior pharnyx. In the unconscious person this is to be expected.

7. ANS—A *IEC—172*

Snoring is best corrected by repositioning the head. If you do not suspect your patient having a cervical spine injury, use the head-tilt chin lift method. In the trauma patient, when cervical spine integrity is compromised, use the modified jaw thrust.

8. ANS—D *IEC—172*

High-pitched "crowing sounds" caused by obstruction of the upper airway are called "stridor." These sounds indicate severe obstruction in the upper airway and are very difficult to correct in the field. Suspect a foreign body or tissue swelling phenomenon.

Chapter 6: General Patient Assessment and Initial Management

9. ANS—A *IEC—172*

The whistling sounds indicative of lower airway obstruction are called "wheezes." These are whistling-type breath sounds associated with narrowing or spasm of the smaller airways.

10. ANS—D *IEC—172*

If your patient presents unconscious without a gag reflex and moving less than 6 liters per minute of air, you should first perform bag-valve mask ventilations with 100% oxygen and plan to intubate the patient.

11. ANS—A *IEC—172*

Normal circulatory status is evidenced by warm, dry skin, the presence of a radial pulse at a rate of 60–100 per minute and capillary refill time of less than 2 seconds.

12. ANS—A *IEC—177*

Four common physical exam techniques are inspection, palpation, ausculation, and percussion.

13. ANS—C *IEC—177*

You may choose to evaluate heart sounds by ausculation. Use the bell side of your stethoscope to pick up the closing of the valves and any extraneous sounds. Place the bell lightly over the heart valves at approximately the third intercostal space just left of the sternum.

14. ANS—A *IEC—178*

Percussion evaluates the surface and the tissue beneath by sending a vibration through it. A hollow and vibrating residence heard when percussing the chest indicates the presence of air.

15. ANS—B *IEC—179*

Battle's sign is a black-and-blue discoloration over the mastoid process just behind the ear. This is characteristic of a basilar skull fracture. It is not commonly seen in the prehospital setting because it takes several hours to produce the discoloration.

16. ANS—D *IEC—179*

The halo test is performed by dropping the fluid in question onto a gauze pad or a sheet. If blood and cerebral spinal fluid are mixed, it will yield a characteristic halo or target sign (darker red circles surrounded by a lighter one). This indicates the presence of cerebrospinal spinal fluid in the blood.

17. ANS—D *IEC—180*

Very small or pin-point pupils suggest intoxication from opium derivatives (narcotics, heroin, morphine, percodan, darvon, codeine).

18. ANS—B *IEC—180*

Failure of the eyes to rotate simultaneously in the same direction is called dysconjugate gaze. This may indicate a pre-existing problem, occular muscle intrapment, or optic nerve damage. Do not attempt this maneuver on any patient with suspected spine injury.

19. _____	Coffee grounds	C. Bleeding in the stomach		*IEC—181*
20. _____	Fresh blood	E. Upper GI hemorrhage		
21. _____	Pink-tinged sputum	A. Congestive heart failure		
22. _____	Green or yellow phlegm	B. Respiratory infection		
23. _____	Vomit	D. Brainstem problem		

24. ANS—B *IEC—182*

You should always examine the jugular veins for distention. In the supine normotensive patient, they should distend slightly. However, as the body is brought to a 45° angle they empty. Distention beyond 45° is indicative of pathology.

25. ANS—C *IEC—182*

Significant jugular venous distention is indicative of cardiac tamponade, tension pneumothorax, right heart failure, or corpulmonale.

26. ANS—C *IEC—182*

If the veins do not distend in the supine position, hypovolemia is the probable cause.

27. ANS—B *IEC—183*

Subcutaneous emphysema is the presence of air within the subcutaneous tissues often associated with pneumothorax. Palpating the skin in this area will produce a crackling sound and feeling.

28. ANS—D *IEC—185*

A rapid, deep respiratory pattern could be due to head injury (central neurogenic hyperventilation), a metabolic problem (diabetic coma), extreme exertion, or hyperventilation syndrome.

29. ANS—D *IEC—185*

Cheyne-Stokes is a respiratory pattern characterized by progressive increase in the rate and volume of respirations that later gradually subside. It is usually associated with a disturbance in the respiratory center of the brain.

30. ANS—B *IEC—186*

Cullen's sign is a bluish discoloration of the area around the umbilicus caused by intra-abdominal hemorrhage.

31. ANS—A *IEC—186*

Rebound tenderness is a physical finding of tenderness upon sudden release of an examining hand from the abdomen often associated with peritoneal irritation.

32. ANS—D *IEC—186*

Ascites is an accumulation of fluid within the abdominal cavity. It is often caused by increased pressure in the systemic circulation (right heart failure) or in the portal system (cirrhosis of the liver). It is associated with congestive heart failure and alcoholism among other causes.

33. ANS—A *IEC—187*

Presacral edema is an accumulation of fluid in flank area in the recumbent patient. This is usually related to congestive heart failure.

34. ANS—D *IEC—187*

Priapism is a painful prolonged erection of the penis. It results from unopposed parasympathetic stimulation. It occurs with spinal cord interruption or certain types of brain dysfunction.

35. ANS—A *IEC—189*

Clubbing is an enlargement of the distal fingers and toes, often due to chronic respiratory or cardiovascular disease.

36. ANS—D *IEC—193*

The difference between systolic and diastolic blood pressures is known as pulse pressure. The patient with a blood pressure of 120/80 has a pulse pressure of 40.

37. ANS—B *IEC—193*

If your supine patient's pulse rate rises more than 15 beats per minute when you sit him up, you should suspect a significant blood loss. This is known as a positive "tilt test," or orthostatic hypotension.

38. ANS—D *IEC—195*

Patients with effective respirations should measure an oxygen saturation of 96–100%. If respirations are compromised even slightly, oxygen saturation falls. Provide any patient whose saturation is below 90% with aggressive oxygenation and possibly positive pressure ventilation.

39. ANS—D *IEC—195*

Pulse oximeter measures the oxygen saturation level of blood through a noninvasive sensor placed on a finger or ear lobe. In low flow states, such as hypothermia and late hypovolemia, the device may not sense accurately. The presence of a carbon monoxide on the hemoglobin molecule tends to elevate the saturation level falsely.

40. ANS—C *IEC—197*

The primary presenting symptom noticed by the patient is called the chief complaint. It is the reason that caused your patient to request help.

41. ANS—B *IEC—197*

When describing your patient's symptoms, it is best to use the patient's own words. In other words, your patient is "having trouble breathing," not "dyspneic."

42. ANS—D *IEC—198*

Referred pain is pain that is referred to other parts of the body. The two most common areas that produce referred pain are the heart and the diaphragm. Pain from the heart is most commonly referred to the left arm. The pain associated with diaphragmatic irritation is generally referred to the clavical region.

43. ANS—C *IEC—200*

The P in AMPLE stands for past medical history.

44. ANS—A *IEC—200*

The M in AMPLE stands for medications taken.

45. ANS—A *IEC—200*

The A in AMPLE stands for allergies.

CHAPTER 7

Advanced Airway Management and Ventilation

QUESTIONS

1. Which of the following is a responsibility of the nasal cavity?
   A. Filter the incoming air.
   B. Humidify the incoming air.
   C. Warm the incoming air.
   D. All of the above.

2. What purpose do the choncae serve?
   A. They secrete mucus into the nasal cavity.
   B. They propel foreign particles into the pharynx.
   C. They cause air flow turbulence.
   D. They stimulate the cilia.

3. The muscular tube that extends from the back of the soft palate to the esophagus is the:
   A. trachea.
   B. larynx.
   C. pharynx.
   D. eustachian tube.

4. A leaf-shaped cartilage that prevents food from entering the larynx during swallowing is the:
   A. arytenoid.
   B. cricoids.
   C. epiglottis.
   D. hyoid.

5. The depression between the epiglottis and the base of the tongue is the:
   A. eustachian tube.
   B. vallecula.

C. hyoid.
D. pyriform fossa.

6. The narrowest part of the adult upper airway is at the level of the:
   A. vocal cords.
   B. cricoid cartilage.
   C. cricothyroid membrane.
   D. hyoid bone.

7. The space between the vocal cords is known as the:
   A. eustachian tube.
   B. hyoid process.
   C. cricothyroid membrane.
   D. glottis.

8. The trachea divides into the right and left mainstem bronchi at the:
   A. hyoid bone.
   B. carina.
   C. vallecula.
   D. parenchyma.

9. An endotracheal tube inserted too far will most likely rest in the:
   A. right mainstem bronchus.
   B. left mainstem bronchus.
   C. lung parenchyma.
   D. carina.

10. Most gas exchange occurs in the:
    A. respiratory bronchioles.
    B. alveoli.
    C. alveolar ducts.
    D. bronchioles.

11. The _____ pleura covers the lungs.
    A. visceral
    B. parietal
    C. pulmonary
    D. respiratory

12. During inspiration, air enters the lungs because of a/an _____ in intrathoracic pressure.
    A. increase
    B. decrease

13. The lungs receive deoxygenated blood from the:
    A. right heart.
    B. left heart.
    C. pulmonary veins.
    D. bronchial arteries.

14. The normal PaO_2 for a healthy adult breathing room air is _____ torr.
    A. 60.
    B. 80–100.
    C. 35–45.
    D. 40.

15. The normal PaCO$_2$ for a healthy adult breathing room air is _____ _____ torr.
   A. 60–80
   B. 80–100
   C. 35–45
   D. 7.35–7.45

16. Oxygen molecules move from the alveoli into the pulmonary capillary because of a process known as:
   A. osmosis.
   B. ventilation/perfusion mismatch.
   C. atelectasis.
   D. diffusion.

17. Ninety-seven percent of the oxygen that enters the bloodstream:
   A. is dissolved in plasma.
   B. binds with hemoglobin.
   C. is transported as bicarbonate.
   D. is exhaled into the atmosphere.

18. In which of the following cases would the oxygen saturation and partial pressure be high yet the patient die of hypoxia?
   A. Carbon monoxide poisoning.
   B. Hypothermia.
   C. Hypovolemia.
   D. All of the above.

19. Which of the following conditions might cause a ventilation/perfusion mismatch?
   A. Pneumothorax.
   B. Hemothorax.
   C. Pulmonary embolism.
   D. All of the above.

20. The FiO$_2$ of room air is:
   A. 80–100 torr.
   B. 21%.
   C. 100%.
   D. 40 torr.

21. When it enters the bloodstream, the majority of carbon dioxide:
   A. is dissolved in plasma.
   B. binds with hemoglobin.
   C. is transported as bicarbonate.
   D. combines with carbon monoxide.

22. Which of the following would **NOT** increase a patient's PaCO$_2$?
   A. Hyperventilation.
   B. Hypoventilation.
   C. Airway obstruction.
   D. Muscle exertion.

23. The main respiratory center lies in the:
   A. apneustic center.
   B. pneumotaxic center.

C. stretch receptors.
D. medulla.

24. The Hering-Breuer Reflex is a process that:
    A. ensures rhythmic inspiration.
    B. monitors for changes in $PaCO_2$.
    C. prevents overinflation of the lungs.
    D. controls hypoxic drive.

25. Chemoreceptors are stimulated by which of the following:
    A. increased PaO_2.
    B. increased $PaCO_2$.
    C. increased pH.
    D. none of the above.

26. Patients with hypoxic drive are stimulated to breathe by:
    A. increases in PaO_2.
    B. decreases in $PaCO_2$.
    C. increases in pH.
    D. none of the above.

Match the following modified forms of respiration with their descriptions:

27. _____ Coughing   A. Prolonged exhalation
28. _____ Sneezing   B. Respiratory distress sign in infants
29. _____ Hiccoughing   C. Protective airway function
30. _____ Sighing   D. Caused by nasal irritation
31. _____ Grunting   E. Diaphragmatic spasm

32. The average volume of gas inhaled in one respiratory cycle is known as:
    A. minute volume.
    B. tidal volume.
    C. alveolar volume.
    D. none of the above.

33. Maximum lung capacity in the average adult male is approximately:
    A. 4500 ml.
    B. 350 ml.
    C. 6000 ml.
    D. 500 ml.

34. The average tidal volume in the healthy adult male is approximately:
    A. 150 ml.
    B. 500 ml.
    C. 350 ml.
    D. 6000 ml.

35. Minute volume is calculated:
    A. respiratory rate × dead air space.
    B. tidal volume − dead air space.
    C. alveolar volume ÷ dead air space.
    D. tidal volume × respiratory rate.

36. The stiffness or flexibility of the lungs is known as:
  A. capnography.
  B. compliance.
  C. saturation.
  D. atelectasis.

37. Upper airway obstruction can be caused by:
  A. anaphylaxis.
  B. epiglottitis.
  C. respiratory burns.
  D. all of the above.

38. Sellick's maneuver is used to:
  A. prevent regurgitation.
  B. aid in EOA insertion.
  C. open the airway in trauma.
  D. all of the above.

39. Your patient is semi-conscious with a gag reflex. Which of the following airway adjuncts is indicated?
  A. Oropharyngeal Airway.
  B. Nasopharyngeal Airway.
  C. Endotracheal tube.
  D. Esophageal Obturator Airway.

40. The major advantage of using a nasopharyngeal airway is that:
  A. it isolates the trachea.
  B. it is easy to suction through.
  C. it can be used in the presence of a gag reflex.
  D. none of the above.

41. The distal cuff on an endotracheal tube should be filled with _____ ml of air.
  A. 5–10.
  B. 10–20.
  C. 20–30.
  D. 30–35.

42. Noncuffed endotracheal tubes are recommended for children under the age of:
  A. 5 years.
  B. 8 years.
  C. 10 years.
  D. 12 years.

43. Endotracheal intubation may be attempted in all of the following situations **EXCEPT**:
  A. patients without a gag reflex.
  B. anaphylaxis.
  C. respiratory burns.
  D. epiglottitis.

44. Which of the following drugs may **NOT** be administered down the endotracheal tube?
  A. Epinephrine.

B. Atropine.
C. Lidocaine.
D. Sodium Bicarbonate.

45. Each endotracheal intubation attempt should be limited to _____ seconds.
A. 10.
B. 15.
C. 30.
D. 60.

46. The endotracheal tube may be misplaced into which of the following structures?
A. Esophagus.
B. Pyriform sinus.
C. Vallecula.
D. All of the above.

47. Which of the following indicates an esophageal intubation?
A. Phonation.
B. Absence of breath sounds.
C. Gurgling sounds heard over the epigastrium.
D. All of the above.

48. The proper position of the head and neck for endotracheal intubation in the non-trauma patient is the _____ position.
A. neutral.
B. hyperextended.
C. sniffing.
D. flexed.

49. The curved, or Macintosh, blade is designed to:
A. lift the epiglottitis.
B. spread the vocal cords.
C. fit into the vallecula.
D. none of the above.

50. If your intubated patient has breath sounds only over the right chest, you should:
A. remove the tube immediately.
B. secure the tube in place.
C. bring the tube back a few centimeters and recheck.
D. push the tube in a few centimeters and recheck.

51. Which of the following is true regarding suctioning?
A. It should be limited to 30 seconds.
B. Apply suction during insertion and during removal.
C. Hyperventilate the patient before and after suctioning.
D. All of the above.

52. The nasal cannula delivers oxygen concentrations in the range of:
A. 10–50%.
B. 50–100%.
C. 24–44%.
D. 40–60%.

Chapter 7: Advanced Airway Management and Ventilation

53. Nasal cannula flow rates should not exceed _____ lpm.
   A. 3.
   B. 6.
   C. 8.
   D. 10.

54. The simple face mask delivers oxygen concentrations in the range of:
   A. 20–40%.
   B. 40–60%.
   C. 60–80%.
   D. 80–100%.

55. Simple face mask flow rates should never fall below _____ lpm.
   A. 3.
   B. 6.
   C. 8.
   D. 10.

56. The nonrebreather mask delivers oxygen concentrations in the range of:
   A. 20–40%.
   B. 40–60%.
   C. 60–80%.
   D. 80–100%.

57. Nonrebreather mask flow rates should never fall below _____ lpm.
   A. 3.
   B. 6.
   C. 8.
   D. 10.

58. The Venturi system delivers oxygen concentrations in the range of:
   A. 24–40%.
   B. 40–60%.
   C. 60–80%.
   D. 80–100%.

59. To achieve effective ventilatory support you must deliver at least _____ _____ ml of oxygen at a rate of _____ breaths per minute.
   A. 300, 16–20.
   B. 500, 12–22.
   C. 800, 12–20.
   D. 1000, 16–24.

60. Using a pocket mask without supplemental oxygen delivers oxygen in the range of:
   A. 16–17%.
   B. 21–22 %.
   C. 20–50%.
   D. 90–100%.

61. A bag-valve-mask device with an oxygen reservoir can deliver up to _____ of oxygen with flow rates at 10–15 lpm.
   A. 50%.
   B. 60%.
   C. 80%.
   D. 95%.

Chapter 7: Advanced Airway Management and Ventilation

62. A demand valve resuscitator will deliver up to _____ oxygen at its highest flow rates.
   A. 50%.
   B. 60%.
   C. 80%.
   D. 100%.

63. Which of the following complications is associated with demand valve use?
   A. pneumothorax.
   B. subcutaneous emphysema.
   C. gastric distention.
   D. all of the above.

64. Which of the following is true regarding the use of an automatic ventilator?
   A. They deliver higher minute volumes than the bag-valve-mask.
   B. Most units deliver controlled ventilation only.
   C. They can be used safely in all age groups.
   D. The pop-off valves should be disengaged.

65. In which of the following cases might higher airway pressures be necessary to ventilate the lungs?
   A. Cardiogenic pulmonary edema.
   B. Adult Respiratory Distress Syndrome.
   C. Bronchospasm.
   D. All of the above.

ANSWERS

1. ANS—D *IEC—172*

The nasal cavity is responsible for filtering, humidifying, and warming the incoming air.

2. ANS—C *IEC—172*

The conchae or turbinates are shelf-like structures that cause turbulent airflow. This turbulence helps deposit any airborne particles onto the mucus membrane that lines the nasal cavity.

3. ANS—C *IEC—173*

The pharynx, or throat, is a muscular tube that extends vertically from the back of the soft palate to the upper end of the esophagus. It allows the flow of air into and out of the respiratory tract and the passage of foods and liquids into the digestive system.

4. ANS—C *IEC—174*

The epiglottis is a leaf-shaped cartilage that prevents food from entering the respiratory tract during the act of swallowing.

5. ANS—B *IEC—174*

The depression between the epiglottis and the base of the tongue is known as the vallecula. This landmark is significant because during intubation, you insert the curved blade into this crevice.

6. ANS—A *IEC—174*

In adults the portion of the thyroid cartilage housing the vocal cords is the narrowest part of the upper airways.

7. ANS—D *IEC—175*

The glottis is the slit-like opening between the vocal cords, also known as the glottic opening.

8. ANS—B *IEC—176*

The carina is the point at which the trachea bifurcates into the right and left mainstem bronchi.

9. ANS—A *IEC—176*

The right mainstem bronchus is almost straight and slightly curved whereas the left main bronchus angles more acutely to the left. An endotracheal tube inserted too far will most likely rest in the right mainstem bronchus for that reason.

10. ANS—B *IEC—177*

A limited gas exchange may occur in the alveolar ducts and respiratory bronchioles. Most gas exchange takes place in the alveoli. The alveoli comprise the key functional unit of the respiratory system.

11. ANS—A *IEC—177*

Lungs are covered by connective tissue called pleura. The pleura consists of two layers; the visceral pleura covers the lungs and does not contain nerve fibers.

12. ANS—B *IEC—178*

During inspiration the size of the thoracic cavity is made larger by contracting the diaphragm and the intercostal muscles. This causes a great and instant decrease in the intrathoracic pressure. This decrease in intrathoracic pressure causes air to rush into the lungs.

13. ANS—A *IEC—178*

The lungs receive deoxygenated blood from the right side of the heart through the pulmonary artery. The pulmonary artery is the only artery in the body that carries deoxygenated blood.

14. ANS—B *IEC—180*

The normal PaO_2 for a healthy adult breathing room air is 80–100 torr.

15. ANS—C *IEC—180*

The normal $PaCO_2$ for a healthy adult breathing room air is 35–45 torr.

16. ANS—D *IEC—181*

Diffusion is the movement of gas from an area of higher partial pressure concentration to an area of lower partial pressure concentration. This process allows oxygen molecules to move from the alveoli into the pulmonary capillary.

17. ANS—B *IEC—180*

Of the oxygen that enters the bloodstream, 97% of it binds with the hemoglobin molecule on the red blood cells. Three percent is dissolved in plasma.

18. ANS—A *IEC—181*

Consider the patient with carbon monoxide poisoning. Since carbon monoxide has a greater affinity for the hemoglobin molecule than oxygen does, it will replace it, if present. That means that most of the oxygen inhaled will be dissolved in plasma. If arterial blood gas samples were taken, it would reveal a normal or high PaO_2 because the PaO_2 measures the freely dissolved oxygen in

48 Chapter 7: Advanced Airway Management and Ventilation

the bloodstream. The pulse oximeter measures the saturation of the hemoglobin molecule. In this case, it is saturated not with oxygen but with carbon monoxide. Both measurements would read high yet the patient would die of hypoxia. It's the hemoglobin that transports oxygen to the peripheral tissues.

19. ANS—D *IEC—181*

Ideally, each milliliter of air we inhale should meet up with 1 ml of blood. When it doesn't, a ventilation/perfusion mismatch occurs. This can be caused by a problem with ventilation or a problem with circulation. Ventilation-perfusion mismatches are the most common cause of respiratory distress.

20. ANS—B *IEC—181*

The FiO_2 is a measurement of the concentration of oxygen in the inspired air. The FiO_2 of room air is approximately .21 (21%).

21. ANS—C *IEC—181*

Carbon dioxide is transported mainly in the form of bicarbonate. Approximately 66% is transported in this manner while 33% is transported combined with hemoglobin. Less than 1% is dissolved in the plasma.

22. ANS—A *IEC—181*

Carbon dioxide concentrations in the blood are influenced by increases and decreases in CO_2 production and/or elimination. $PaCO_2$ would be increased by hypoventilation, airway obstruction, or muscle exertion.

23. ANS—D *IEC—182*

The respiratory center lies in the medulla located in the brain stem.

24. ANS—C *IEC—182*

The Hering-Breuer reflex is a process that prevents over-expansion of the lungs. During inspiration the lungs become distended activating what are known as stretch receptors. As the degree of stretch increases, these receptors fire more frequently sending a message to the brain stem to inhibit the respiratory inspiration.

25. ANS—B *IEC—182*

Receptors are located in the carotid bodies, the aortic arch, and in the medulla. In the normal person these chemoreceptors are stimulated by decreased PaO_2, increased $PaCO_2$, and a decreased pH.

26. ANS—D *IEC—183*

People with chronic respiratory disease such as emphysema and chronic bronchitis tend to retain carbon dioxide and often develop a condition known as hypoxic drive. These patients are stimulated to breath by decreases in PaO_2.

27. _____	Coughing	**C.**	Protective airway function	*IEC—183*
28. _____	Sneezing	**D.**	Caused by nasal irritation	
29. _____	Hiccoughing	**E.**	Diaphragmatic spasm	
30. _____	Sighing	**A.**	Prolonged exhalation	
31. _____	Grunting	**B.**	Respiratory distress sign in infants	

32. ANS—B *IEC—185*

Tidal volume is the average volume of gas inhaled or exhaled in one respiratory cycle.

33. ANS—C *IEC—185*

Total lung capacity in the average adult male is approximately six liters.

Chapter 7: Advanced Airway Management and Ventilation   **49**

34. ANS—B *IEC—185*

The average tidal volume in a healthy adult male is approximately 500 ml.

35. ANS—D *IEC—185*

Minute volume is the amount of gas moved in and out of the respiratory tract in one minute. It is measured by multiplying the tidal volume times the respiratory rate.

36. ANS—B *IEC—191*

Compliance refers to the stiffness or flexibility of the lung tissue. It is determined by how easily air flows into the lungs. When compliance is good, airflow occurs with a minimal amount of resistance. Poor compliance means that ventilation is harder to achieve. It is often poor in diseased lungs, patients with chest wall injuries, or tension pneumothorax.

37. ANS—D *IEC—186*

Upper airway obstruction can be caused by anaphylaxis, epiglottitis, and respiratory burns.

38. ANS—A *IEC—196*

Sellick's maneuver is used to prevent regurgitation by applying slight pressure posteriorly over the cricoid cartilage thus closing off the esophagus. It is also useful in endotracheal intubation to help bring the larynx into view.

39. ANS—B *IEC—200*

In the semi-conscious patient with a gag reflex, the nasopharyngeal airway is an excellent initial airway adjunct.

40. ANS—C *IEC—200*

The major advantage of using the nasopharyngeal airway is that it can be used in the presence of the gag reflex.

41. ANS—A *IEC—210*

The cuff of an endotracheal tube should be filled with 5-10 ml of air.

42. ANS—B *IEC—210*

Non-cuffed endotracheal tubes are recommended for children under the age of 8 years old. In these children the cricoid cartilage acts as an anatomical cuff since it is the narrowest part of the pediatric airway.

43. ANS—D *IEC—213*

Tracheal intubation should never be attempted in patients suspected of having epiglottis. Any unnecessary agitation of the patient can cause immediate laryngospasm and subsequent respiratory arrest.

44. ANS—D *IEC—214*

The following medications can be administered down the endotracheal tube: oxygen, naloxone, atropine, diazepam, epinephrine, lidocaine. Just remember O-NAVEL.

45. ANS—C *IEC—215*

According to the American Heart Association, endotracheal intubation attempts should be limited to no more than 30 seconds to prevent hypoxia.

46. ANS—D *IEC—215*

The endotracheal tube may be misplaced into the esophagus, the pyriform sinus, or the vallecula.

47. ANS—D *IEC—215*

Signs of an esophageal intubation include an absence of chest rise and breath sounds with ventilatory support; gurgling sounds heard over the epigastrium; the absence of breath condensation in the endotracheal tube; a persistent air leak despite inflation of the distal cuff; cyanosis; progressive worsening of the patient's condition; and phonation.

48. ANS—C *IEC—216*

The proper position of the head and neck for endotracheal intubation in the non-trauma patient is the sniffing position. This is accomplished by flexing the neck forward and the head backward or by inserting a roll towel under the patient's shoulders or the back of the head.

49. ANS—C *IEC—216*

The curved, or Macintosh, blade is designed to fit into the vallecula. The vallecula is the space between the base of the tongue and the epiglottis.

50. ANS—C *IEC—217*

If your intubated patient has breath sounds heard only over the right chest, you should assume a right mainstem bronchus intubation. In this case, withdraw the tube back a few centimeters and recheck placement.

51. ANS—C *IEC—243*

Suctioning should always be limited to 15 seconds. You should hyperventilate the patient before and after all suctioning attempts and always apply suction during removal.

52. ANS—C *IEC—247*

The nasal cannula delivers oxygen concentrations in the range of 24–44% depending on the liter flow.

NASAL CANNULA OXYGEN DELIVERY	
Liter Flow	*Approximate Oxygen Concentration Delivered*
1	24
2	28
3	32
4	36
5	40
6	44

53. ANS—B *IEC—246*

Nasal cannulla flow rates should not exceed 6 liters per minute as this will dry the mucus membrane and cause headaches.

54. ANS—B *IEC—247*

The simple face mask delivers oxygen concentrations in the range of 40–60%. Oxygen is delivered through the bottom of the mask via its oxygen inlet port.

55. ANS—B *IEC—248*

No fewer than 6 liters per minute should be administered through this device as expired carbon dioxide can otherwise accumulate in the mask.

Chapter 7: Advanced Airway Management and Ventilation **51**

56. ANS—D *IEC—248*

The nonrebreather mask consists of oxygen tubing and a face mask with an attached reservoir bag. When the patient inhales, 100% oxygen contained in the reservoir is drawn into the mask and the patient's respiratory passageways. The nonrebreather mask delivers the highest concentration of oxygen. Once applied a flowrate of 10–15 liters per minute can deliver an 80–100% oxygen concentration.

57. ANS—D *IEC—249*

No fewer than 8 liters of oxygen per minute should be administered through this device.

58. ANS—A *IEC—249*

The venturi system is a high flow device including oxygen tubing, a face mask, and the venturi system. As oxygen passes through a jet port in the base of the mask, it entrains room air. Depending on the device used, oxygen concentrations can be delivered in the range of 24–40%.

59. ANS—C *IEC—250*

To achieve adequate ventilatory support, you must deliver at least 800 ml of oxygen at a rate of 12–20 breaths per minute.

60. ANS—A *IEC—251*

Using a pocket mask without supplemental oxygen delivers the oxygen in the range of 16–17%. In other words, your own expired FiO_2.

61. ANS—D *IEC—251*

A bag-valve mask device with an oxygen reservoir can deliver up to 95% of oxygen with flow rates at 10–15 liters per minute.

62. ANS—D *IEC—252*

A demand valve resuscitator will deliver up to 100% oxygen at its highest flow rates.

63. ANS—D *IEC—252*

Using a demand valve has its disadvantages. Some of these include creating a pneumothorax, subcutaneous emphysema, or gastric distension.

64. ANS—A *IEC—253*

Automatic ventilators deliver higher minute volumes than the bag-valve mask.

65. ANS—D *IEC—253*

In cases such as cardiodemic pulmonary edema, adult respiratory distress syndrome, and bronchospasm, higher airway pressures may be necessary to ventilate the lungs.

CHAPTER 8

Fluids and Shock

QUESTIONS

1. Water makes up approximately _____ of total body weight.
    A. 30%
    B. 60%
    C. 80%
    D. none of the above

2. Where is most of this water found?
    A. Between the cells.
    B. In the blood vessels.
    C. In the cells.
    D. None of the above.

3. All of the following happens when your fluid levels drop **EXCEPT:**
    A. ADH is secreted.
    B. the kidneys reabsorb sodium.
    C. more urine is excreted.
    D. water shifts into the intravascular compartment.

4. All of the following are signs of dehydration **EXCEPT:**
    A. poor skin turgor.
    B. sacral edema.
    C. sunken fontanelles.
    D. tachycardia.

5. Dehydrated patients should receive:
    A. an isotonic solution.
    B. Lactated Ringer's.
    C. normal saline.
    D. all of the above.

6. A medication that stimulates the kidneys to excrete water is a/an:
   A. cation.
   B. anion.
   C. diuretic.
   D. homeostatic.

7. A positively charged ion is called a/an:
   A. cation.
   B. anion.
   C. colloid.
   D. crystalloid.

8. The chief extracellular cation that regulates fluid distribution is:
   A. bicarbonate.
   B. sodium.
   C. potassium.
   D. magnesium.

9. The chief intracellular cation that aids in electrical impulse transmission is:
   A. magnesium.
   B. sodium.
   C. potassium.
   D. calcium.

10. The cation that plays a major role in muscle contraction is:
    A. bicarbonate.
    B. sodium.
    C. potassium.
    D. calcium.

11. The principle buffer of the acid-base system is:
    A. bicarbonate.
    B. sodium.
    C. potassium.
    D. magnesium.

12. Electrolytes are measured in:
    A. mg/kg.
    B. mEq/L.
    C. mEq/dl.
    D. mcg/L.

13. The movement of water through a semi-permeable membrane from an area of low solute concentration toward an area of high solute concentration is called:
    A. diffusion.
    B. facilitated diffusion.
    C. active transport.
    D. osmosis.

14. Infusing a hypotonic solution into the bloodstream will cause water to move in the following direction:
    A. into the cells.
    B. into the blood vessel.

C. out of the cells.
D. none of the above.

15. The movement of solute particles through a semi-permeable membrane from an area of high solute concentration toward an area of low solute concentration is called:
A. diffusion.
B. facilitated diffusion.
C. active transport.
D. osmosis.

16. Infusing a hypertonic solution into a blood vessel will cause all of the following to happen EXCEPT:
A. an osmotic gradient toward the vein.
B. a fluid shift into the blood vessel.
C. an increase in blood pressure.
D. a decrease in intravascular blood volume.

17. A solution with the same osmolarity as blood plasma is said to be:
A. hypotonic.
B. hypertonic.
C. isotonic.
D. none of the above.

18. In a fresh water drowning, what happens as water enters the pulmonary capillaries?
A. It remains in the capillaries.
B. It quickly diffuses into the cells.
C. It draws additional fluid into the blood vessel.
D. None of the above.

19. Sodium is transported out of the cell against the gradient in a process called:
A. facilitated diffusion.
B. facilitated transport.
C. passive diffusion.
D. active transport.

20. The insulin/glucose relationship is an example of:
A. facilitated diffusion.
B. facilitated transport.
C. passive diffusion.
D. active transport.

21. The majority of blood volume consists of:
A. red blood cells.
B. plasma.
C. platelets.
D. white blood cells.

22. The percentage of red blood cells in the blood is called:
A. homeostasis.
B. hematocrit.
C. hemoglobin.
D. hematoma.

23. Red blood cells make up what percentage of total blood volume in the healthy adult?
  A. 20.
  B. 45.
  C. 55.
  D. 60.

24. The universal recipient is blood type:
  A. A.
  B. B.
  C. AB.
  D. O.

25. The universal donor is blood type:
  A. A.
  B. B.
  C. AB.
  D. O.

26. A patient with blood infusing suddenly develops fever, chills, nausea, hives, tachycardia, and hypotension. You suspect a transfusion reaction. Which of the following should you do?
  A. Stop the IV.
  B. Infuse normal saline.
  C. Monitor the patient closely.
  D. All of the above.

27. Hespan, Dextran, and Albumin are examples of:
  A. colloids.
  B. crystalloids.
  C. isotonic solutions.
  D. hypotonic solutions.

28. After infusing a colloid solution, you should expect:
  A. a decrease in blood pressure.
  B. a fluid shift into the bloodstream.
  C. rapid diffusion of its solute particles into the tissues.
  D. an osmotic gradient toward the intracellular compartment.

29. How much Lactated Ringer's solution remains in the intravascular compartment after one hour?
  A. 100%.
  B. 66%.
  C. 50%.
  D. 33%.

30. The normal pH for the human body is:
  A. 7.0–8.0.
  B. 7.35–7.45.
  C. 7.3.
  D. 7.5.

31. The fastest mechanism for correcting the body's acid-base abnormalities is the:
  A. respiratory system.

B. renal system.
C. buffer system.
D. none of the above.

32. A patient with a pH of 7.2 and a PaCO$_2$ of 52 torr is in a state of:
A. respiratory acidosis.
B. respiratory alkalosis.
C. metabolic acidosis.
D. metabolic alkalosis.

33. A probable cause of this patient's condition is:
A. near drowning.
B. amphetamine drug overdose.
C. antacid ingestion.
D. excessive vomiting.

34. The reasons behind the pH and PaCO$_2$ abnormalities include:
A. an increase in carbon dioxide elimination.
B. an increase in bicarbonate concentration.
C. a decrease in carbon dioxideretention.
D. none of the above.

35. Immediate management of a patient in respiratory acidosis includes:
A. coaching the patient to breathe slower.
B. administration of sodium bicarbonate.
C. positive pressure ventilation.
D. none of the above.

36. Which of the following is true regarding a patient in alkalosis?
A. The pH is abnormally low.
B. The hydrogen ion concentration is abnormally high.
C. There are no bicarbonate ions present.
D. None of the above.

37. Management of the patient in respiratory alkalosis includes:
A. hyperventilation.
B. coaching and reassurance.
C. breathing into a paper bag.
D. administration of sodium bicarbonate.

38. The chief buffer of the acid-base system is:
A. phosphorus.
B. carbonic acid.
C. bicarbonate.
D. carbonic anhydrase.

39. Which of the following factors **DOES NOT AFFECT** the heart's stroke volume?
A. Heart rate.
B. Preload.
C. Afterload.
D. Contractile force.

40. Preload could be increased by all of the following **EXCEPT:**
A. increasing venous return.
B. increasing contractile force.

C. decreasing afterload.
D. promoting venodilation.

41. The amount of blood pumped from the heart in one contraction is called:
    A. preload.
    B. afterload.
    C. stroke volume.
    D. tidal volume.

42. Which of the following statements best illustrates the Frank-Starling mechanism?
    A. The greater the afterload, the greater the stroke volume.
    B. The less stroke volume, the less the afterload.
    C. The greater the preload, the greater the stroke volume.
    D. The less preload, the greater the afterload.

43. In order to decrease the workload on the heart in a patient with CHF you should:
    A. place the victim in Trendelenberg.
    B. administer a drug that dilates the veins.
    C. administer a fluid challenge.
    D. hyperventilate the patient.

44. The amount of blood pumped by the heart in one minute is called:
    A. minute volume.
    B. stroke volume.
    C. cardiac output.
    D. contractile volume.

45. The amount of resistance against which the heart must pump in order to eject blood is called:
    A. stroke volume.
    B. end-diastolic volume.
    C. afterload.
    D. pulse pressure.

46. Baroreceptors constantly monitor for changes in:
    A. oxygen levels.
    B. carbon dioxide levels.
    C. heart rate.
    D. blood pressure.

47. Stimulation of the baroreceptors causes all of the following **EXCEPT**:
    A. peripheral vasodilation.
    B. increased cardiac output.
    C. increased heart rate.
    D. bronchodilation.

48. Peripheral vascular resistance is dependent upon:
    A. vessel diameter.
    B. fluid viscosity.
    C. vessel length.
    D. all of the above.

49. The greatest change in peripheral resistance occurs in the:
    A. aorta.
    B. arteries.

C. arterioles.
D. capillaries.

50. Which of the following is a component of the "Fick Principle"?
   A. Adequate FiO_2.
   B. Adequate hematocrit.
   C. Adequate diffusion of gases.
   D. All of the above.

51. Anaerobic metabolism results in which of the following?
   A. Inefficient energy.
   B. Increased pyruvic acid formation.
   C. Glycolysis.
   D. All of the above.

52. Tachycardia, cool, clammy, and pale skin, and a stable blood pressure describes a patient in:
   A. compensated shock.
   B. decompensated shock.
   C. irreversible shock.
   D. none of the above.

53. Which of the following happens in decompensated shock?
   A. Pre-capillary sphinctors open.
   B. Rouleaux formation.
   C. Blood pressure falls.
   D. All of the above.

54. In which of the following situations is the PASG **CONTRAINDICATED**?
   A. Suspected intra-abdominal hemorrhage.
   B. Lower extremity hemorrhage.
   C. Acute pulmonary edema secondary to cardiogenic shock.
   D. Pelvic fracture.

55. In a microdrip solution set, _____ drops equals 1 ml.
   A. 10
   B. 15
   C. 30
   D. 60

56. Through which of the following catheters can you deliver the most rapid fluid challenge?
   A. 12 gauge, 4 inch.
   B. 12 gauge, 1 inch.
   C. 24 gauge, 4 inch.
   D. 24 gauge, 1 inch.

57. Chills, fever, nausea, and vomiting following IV insertion indicates a/an:
   A. inadvertent arterial puncture.
   B. pyrogenic reaction.
   C. thrombophlebitis.
   D. air embolism.

58. In this case you should immediately:
   A. place the patient head down on his left side.
   B. place warm packs on the IV site.

C. stop the IV.
D. clear the IV line of any air.

59. The maximum amount of IV fluids that you should administer in the field is:
A. 1 liter.
B. 2–3 liters.
C. 5 liters.
D. none of the above.

ANSWERS

1. ANS—B *IEC—259*

Water is the most abundant substance in the human body. In fact, it counts for approximately 60% of the total body weight.

2. ANS—C *IEC—259*

Approximately 75% of all body water is found within the intracellular compartment. This compartment is found inside the body's cells.

BODY FLUID COMPARTMENTS		
Compartment	Percentage of Total Body Water	Volume in 70 kg Adult
Intracellular Fluid	75%	31.50 L
Extracellular Fluid	25%	10.50 L
Interstitial Fluid	17.5%	7.35 L
Intravascular Fluid	7.5%	3.15 L

3. ANS—C *IEC—266*

When your fluid levels drop, the pituitary gland at the base of the brain secretes the hormone ADH, or antidiuretic hormone. ADH causes the kidneys to reabsorb more water back into the bloodstream and excrete less urine.

4. ANS—B *IEC—267*

Clinically, the dehydrated patient exhibits dry mucous membranes and poor skin turgor. As the dehydration becomes more severe, the pulse will quicken, and the blood pressure will drop. In infants, the anterior fontenal may be sunken.

5. ANS—D *IEC—267*

Treatment for dehydration is fluid replacement. Since you cannot determine electrolyte deficits in the field, you should use isotonic solutions such as normal saline or Lactated Ringer's. For mild to moderate dehydration, run the infusion at 100–200 ml per hour.

6. ANS—C *IEC—268*

The medication that stimulates the kidneys to excrete water is called a diuretic. An example of a diuretic is lasix or furosemide.

7. ANS—A *IEC—260*

Electrolytes are substances that dissociate into charged particles when placed into water. Ions with a positive charge are called cations.

8. ANS—B *IEC—261*

Sodium is the most prevalent cation in the extracellular fluid. It plays a major role in regulating the distribution of water.

9. ANS—C *IEC—261*

Potassium is the most prevalent cation in the intracellular fluid. It plays an important role in the transmission of electrical impulses.

10. ANS—D *IEC—261*

Calcium has many physiological functions. It plays a major role in muscular contraction as well as nerve impulse transmission.

11. ANS—A *IEC—261*

Bicarbonate is the principal buffer of the body. It neutralizes the highly acidic hydrogen ion and other organic acids.

12. ANS—B *IEC—261*

Electrolytes are usually measured in milliequivalents per liter—mEq/L.

13. ANS—D *IEC—262*

Osmosis is the movement of water across a semi-permeable membrane from an area of lesser solute concentration to an area of greater solute concentration. This movement occurs until the solute concentrations on both sides are equal.

Figure 8-1

Osmosis

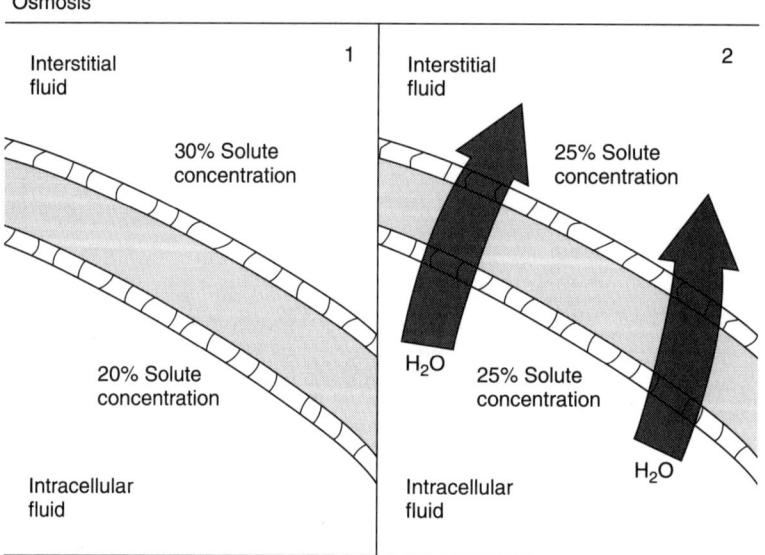

14. ANS—A *IEC—262*

Infusing a hypotonic solution into the bloodstream causes water to move from the bloodstream into the cells. This occurs because water tends to move from areas of low solute concentration, which in this case will be the blood stream, toward areas of higher solute concentration, which in this case will be the interstitial spaces and cells.

15. ANS—A *IEC—262*

Diffusion is the movement of solutes from an area of greater concentration to an area of lesser concentration. This movement occurs until the solute concentrations on both sides are equal.

Figure 8-2
Diffusion

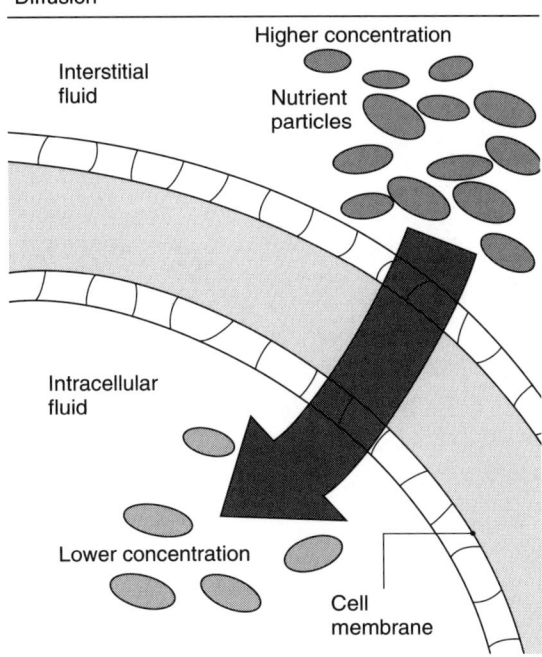

16. ANS—D   *IEC—262*

Infusing a hypertonic solution into a blood vessel will cause an osmotic gradient, which shifts water into the blood vessel. This will cause an increase in blood pressure.

17. ANS—C   *IEC—262*

A solution with the same osmolarity as blood plasma is isotonic. Isotonic is a state in which solutions on opposite sides of a semi-permeable membrane are in equal concentration.

18. ANS—B   *IEC—262*

In a fresh water drowning, water enters the pulmonary capillaries and quickly diffuses into the cells. This occurs because fresh water is hypotonic.

19. ANS—D   *IEC—263*

Sodium is transported out of the cell by a process called active transport. Active transport is a biochemical process in which substances use energy to move across the cell membrane against the normal gradiant. Active transport is faster than diffusion, but it requires the expenditure of energy.

20. ANS—A   *IEC—264*

The insulin-glucose relationship is an example of facilitated diffusion. Facilitated diffusion is a biochemical process in which a substance is selectively transported across a membrane using helper proteins and requires energy.

21. ANS—B   *IEC—264*

Plasma makes up approximately 55% of the total blood volume. It consists of 92% water, 6–7% proteins, and a small portion consisting of electrolytes, lipids, enzymes, clotting factors, glucose, and other dissolved substances.

22. ANS—B   *IEC—265*

The percentage of blood occupied by red blood cells is referred to as the hematocrit. Normal hematocrit in a healthy person is approximately 45%.

23. ANS—B *IEC—264*

Red blood cells account for approximately 45% of the total blood volume. This percentage is known as the patient's hematocrit.

24. ANS—C *IEC—265*

Persons with type AB blood are referred to as universal recipients. These people do not have antibodies to either A or B since they carry both antigens. In an emergency, they can receive blood of any type.

BLOOD TYPING—ABO SYSTEM		
Blood Type	Antigen Present on RBC	Antibody Present in Serum
O	None	Anti-A, Anti-B
AB	A and B	None
B	B	Anti-A
A	A	Anti-B

25. ANS—D *IEC—266*

Type O blood does not contain either the A or B antigen. In an emergency, it can be administered to a patient of any blood type. Because of this, type O is referred to as the universal donor.

COMPATIBILITY AMONG ABO BLOOD GROUPS				
	Reaction with Serum of Recipient			
Cells of Donor	AB	B	A	O
AB	−	+	+	+
B	−	−	+	+
A	−	+	−	+
O	−	−	−	−

− = Nonagglutination
+ = Agglutination

26. ANS—D *IEC—269*

Signs and symptoms of a transfusion reaction include fever, chills, hives, hypotension, palpitations, tachycardia, flushing of the skin, headaches, loss of consciousness, nausea and vomiting, and shortness of breath. If you suspect a transfusion reaction, stop the IV, infuse normal saline, and monitor the patient closely.

27. ANS—A *IEC—269*

Hespan, Dextran, and Albumin are examples of colloids. Colloids are solutions that contain proteins or other high molecular weight molecules that tend to remain in the intravascular space for an extended period of time.

28. ANS—B *IEC—269*

Colloids create a colloid osmotic pressure and tend to attract water into the intravascular space. Colloids draw water from the interstitial spaces and the intracellular compartment in order to increase the intravascular blood volume.

Chapter 8: Fluids and Shock **63**

29. ANS—D *IEC—271*

Due to the movement of the electrolytes and water, two-thirds of crystalloid solutions, such as Lactated Ringer's and normal saline, is lost to the interstitial space within one hour.

30. ANS—B *IEC—272*

The normal pH for the human body is 7.35–7.45.

31. ANS—C *IEC—272*

There are three major mechanisms to remove acids from the body. The fastest mechanism is often referred to as the buffer system, or the bicarbonate buffer system. This system works in seconds.

32. ANS—A *IEC—275*

A patient with a pH of 7.2 and a $PaCO_2$ of 52 torr is in a state of respiratory acidosis.

33. ANS—A *IEC—275*

A probable cause for this patient's condition could be a near-drowning. Respiratory acidosis is caused by the retention of carbon dioxide. This can result from impaired ventilation due to problems occurring in either the lungs or in the respiratory center of the brain.

34. ANS—D *IEC—275*

The reasons behind this patient's pH and PCO_2 levels include a decrease in carbon dioxide elimination and an increase in carbon dioxide retention.

35. ANS—C *IEC—275*

Immediate management of the patient in respiratory acidosis is aimed at improving ventilation and oxygenation. Vigorously ventilate this patient with positive pressure and 100% oxygen.

36. ANS—D *IEC—275*

Alkalosis is a state in which the patient's hyrodgen ion concentration is abnormally low and the pH is high.

37. ANS—B *IEC—275*

Management of a patient in respiratory alkalosis is aimed at helping the patient retain carbon dioxide. Respiratory alkalosis results from the excessive elimination of carbon dioxide. This can occur with anxiety or following climbing to a high altitude. It can also occur as a compensatory mechanism in shock and a variety of other serious hypoxic conditions. For this reason, withholding oxygen from this patient could prove to be a fatal mistake. Simply place your patient on a rebreather mask with 10–15 lpm. oxygen flow and coach him to breathe slowly.

38. ANS—C *IEC—273*

The chief buffer of the acid-base system is bicarbonate.

39. ANS—A *IEC—276*

The amount of blood ejected by the heart at one contraction is referred to as the stroke volume. Stroke volume is determined by preload, afterload, and contractile force.

40. ANS—D *IEC—276*

Preload could be increased by increasing venous return, by increasing contractile force of the heart, and by decreasing the afterload.

41. ANS—C *IEC—276*

The amount of blood pumped from the heart in one contraction is called stroke volume.

42. ANS—C *IEC—277*

The greater the volume of preload, the more the ventricles are stretched. The greater the stretch, up to a certain point, the greater the subsequent cardiac contraction. This is referred to as the Frank-Starling mechanism.

43. ANS—B *IEC—277*

For a patient in severe congestive heart failure, you want to decrease the workload on the heart by decreasing preload. You could accomplish this by administering drugs such as nitroglycerin, furosemide, and morphine, which dilate the veins. Dilating the veins causes pooling of blood on the venous side and decreases preload.

44. ANS—C *IEC—277*

The amount of blood pumped from the heart in one minute is called cardiac output. Cardiac output is calculated by stroke volume times heart rate.

45. ANS—C *IEC—277*

The amount of resistance against which the heart must pump is called afterload. The heart must overcome this resistance in order to eject blood. Afterload is determined by the degree of peripheral vascular resistance. Peripheral resistance is determined by the degree of vasoconstriction present on the arterial side.

46. ANS—D *IEC—278*

Baroreceptors are located in the carotid bodies and the arch of the aorta. These baroreceptors closely monitor pressure.

47. ANS—A *IEC—278*

Baroreceptors are stretch receptors that stretch with increased pressure. When they detect reduced flow and pressure they send messages to the brain to stimulate the sympathetic nervous system. This results in increased heart rate and cardiac output to increase circulation and bronchodilation.

48. ANS—D *IEC—278*

Blood flow through a blood vessel is determined by peripheral resistance and pressure within the system. Peripheral resistance is defined as resistance to blood flow and is dependent upon three factors, the length of the vessel, the diameter of the vessel, and blood viscosity.

49. ANS—C *IEC—278*

There is very little resistance to blood flow through the aorta and arteries. A significant change in peripheral resistance occurs at the arteriole level. This is because the inside diameter of the arteriole is much smaller as compared to the aorta and arteries. Additionally, the arteriole has pronounced ability to change its diameter as much as five-fold in response to local tissue needs and autonomic nervous system signals.

50. ANS—D *IEC—279*

The movement and utilization of oxygen in the body depends upon the following conditions: adequate concentration of inspired oxygen; appropriate movement of oxygen across the alveolar-capillary membrane into the bloodstream; adequate number of red blood cells to carry the oxygen; proper tissue perfusion; and efficient off-loading of oxygen at the tissue level. These conditions are collectively known as the Fick Principle.

51. ANS—D *IEC—280*

During periods of inadequate tissue perfusion, cell metabolism switches from aerobic to an anaerobic mode. Results of this process are inefficient energy, an increase in pyruvic acid formation, and glycoloysis.

52. ANS—A *IEC—281*

Following the onset of inadequate tissue perfusion, various compensatory mechanisms of the body are stimulated. The heart rate and strength of cardiac contractions increase. There will be an increase in systemic vascular resistance to assist in maintaining the blood pressure. These compensatory changes will continue until the body is unable to maintain blood pressure and tissue perfusion. Your patient in compensatory shock will exhibit tachycardia, cool, clammy, and pale skin with a stable blood pressure.

53. ANS—D *IEC—282*

In the later stages of shock the blood pressure begins to fall and blood supply to essential organs diminishes. As a result, the pre-capillary sphinctors open while the post-capillary sphinctors remain closed. This results in sludging of red blood cells and the formation of rouleaux.

54. ANS—C *IEC—305*

Application of the pneumatic anti-shock garment is contraindicated in the presence of pulmonary edema occurring secondary to heart failure. This is because adding fluid volume to the central circulation and increasing afterload may further compromise an already failing heart.

55. ANS—D *IEC—299*

In a microdrip solution set, 60 drops equals 1 ml.

56. ANS—B *IEC—299*

In order to infuse the most fluid most rapidly, use the largest diameter cannula with the shortest possible needle length.

57. ANS—B *IEC—304*

A pyrogenic reaction occurs when pyrogens, "foreign particles capable of producing fever," are present in the administration set or intravenous solution. It is characterized by the abrupt onset of fever, chills, backache, headache, nausea, and vomiting. Cardiovascular collapse may also result.

58. ANS—C *IEC—304*

In a case of pyrogenic reaction, terminate the IV immediately and establish another IV in the other arm using a new administration set and solution.

59. ANS—B *IEC—305*

The maximum amount of intravenous fluids that should be administered to an adult in the field setting is about 2–3 liters. More than 2–3 liters of fluid therapy would reduce the hematocrit to the point of being ineffective.

Appendix

QUESTIONS
1. The great vessels enter the heart through its:
   A. base.
   B. apex.
   C. midline.
   D. ventricles.

2. The innermost layer of the heart, which lines the chambers, is the:
   A. myocardium.
   B. endocardium.
   C. epicardium.
   D. pericardium.

3. The muscular layer of the heart is the:
   A. myocardium.
   B. endocardium.
   C. epicardium.
   D. pericardium.

4. The visceral pericardium is contiguous with the:
   A. myocardium.
   B. endocardium.
   C. epicardium.
   D. pleura.

5. The protective sac surrounding the heart is the:
   A. myocardium.
   B. endocardium.
   C. epicardium.
   D. pericardium.

6. The inferior chambers are the:
   A. atria.
   B. auricles.
   C. ventricles.
   D. vesicles.

7. The only arteries that carry oxygen-poor blood are the:
   A. coronary arteries.
   B. carotid arteries.
   C. mesenteric arteries.
   D. pulmonary arteries.

8. The only veins that carry oxygen-rich blood are the:
   A. vena cava.
   B. pulmonary veins.
   C. coronary veins.
   D. jugular veins.

9. The greatest muscle mass is found in the:
   A. right atrium.
   B. right ventricle.
   C. left atrium.
   D. left ventricle.

10. Which valves are open during systole?
    A. Mitral and tricuspid valves.
    B. Aortic and pulmonic valves.
    C. AV valves.
    D. None of the above.

11. Which valves are open during diastole?
    A. Mitral and tricuspid valves.
    B. Aortic and pulmonic valves.
    C. Semi-lunar valves.
    D. None of the above.

12. The heart muscle is perfused by the:
    A. coronary arteries.
    B. cerebral arteries.
    C. inferior vena cava.
    D. subclavian arteries.

13. The development of collateral circulation is made possible by the presence of:
    A. the coronary sinus.
    B. the aorta.
    C. anastamoses.
    D. automaticity.

14. Blood from the coronary veins empty into the:
    A. right atrium.
    B. left atrium.
    C. right ventricle.
    D. left ventricle.

15. Which of the following does NOT occur during diastole?
    A. Ventricular filling.
    B. Coronary artery perfusion.
    C. AV valves closed.
    D. Atrial contraction.

16. The amount of blood ejected by the heart in one contraction is called:
    A. preload.
    B. cardiac output.
    C. blood pressure.
    D. stroke volume.

17. Up to a point, the greater the venous return to the heart, the greater the:
    A. contractile force.
    B. heart rate.
    C. afterload.
    D. blood pressure.

18. A person with a stroke volume of 70 ml and a heart rate of 80 has a cardiac output of:
    A. 5600 ml.
    B. 1500 ml.
    C. 560 ml.
    D. 150 ml.

19. Specialized structures designed to speed conduction from one muscle fiber to the next are the:
    A. syncytial tissues.
    B. inotropic fibers.
    C. intercalated discs.
    D. autonomic cells.

20. The ventricular syncytium occurs in an inferior to superior direction in order to:
    A. direct blood to the aorta and pulmonary artery.
    B. direct conduction through the AV node.
    C. enhance conduction velocity toward the atria.
    D. avoid the vagus nerve.

21. The normal intrinsic firing rate of the SA node is:
    A. 20–40 beats per minute.
    B. 40–60 beats per minute.
    C. 60–100 beats per minute.
    D. none of the above.

22. The normal intrinsic firing rate of the AV junction is:
    A. 20–40 beats per minute.
    B. 40–60 beats per minute.
    C. 60–100 beats per minute.
    D. none of the above.

23. The normal intrinsic firing rate of the purkinje system is:
    A. 20–40 beats per minute.
    B. 40–60 beats per minute.

C. 60–100 beats per minute.
D. none of the above.

24. Which of the following information can be obtained from a single-lead ECG reading?
   A. The presence of an infarct.
   B. Cardiac output.
   C. Chamber enlargement.
   D. Heart rate.

25. On the vertical axis of a standard ECG graph paper, a deflection of two large boxes signifies:
   A. 1 mV of amplitude.
   B. 10 mV of amplitude.
   C. 0.4 seconds duration.
   D. 2.0 seconds duration.

26. On the horizontal axis of a standard ECG graph paper, a deflection of one large box signifies:
   A. 1 mV of amplitude.
   B. 10 mV of amplitude.
   C. 0.2 seconds duration.
   D. 0.04 seconds duration.

27. The P wave represents:
   A. atrial depolarization.
   B. ventricular depolarization.
   C. delay at the AV node.
   D. ventricular repolarization.

28. The T wave represents:
   A. atrial depolarization.
   B. ventricular depolarization.
   C. delay at the AV node.
   D. ventricular repolarization.

29. The QRS complex represents:
   A. atrial depolarization.
   B. ventricular depolarization.
   C. delay at the AV node.
   D. ventricular repolarization.

30. The P-R interval represents:
   A. atrial depolarization.
   B. ventricular depolarization.
   C. delay at the AV node.
   D. ventricular repolarization.

31. Which of the following may produce artifact on the ECG?
   A. Muscle tremors.
   B. Loose electrodes.
   C. 60 hertz interference.
   D. All of the above.

SCENARIO Your patient is a 45-year-old male who complains of chest pain and shortness of breath. During your work-up he suddenly becomes unconscious and slumps over. His EKG changes are as follows:

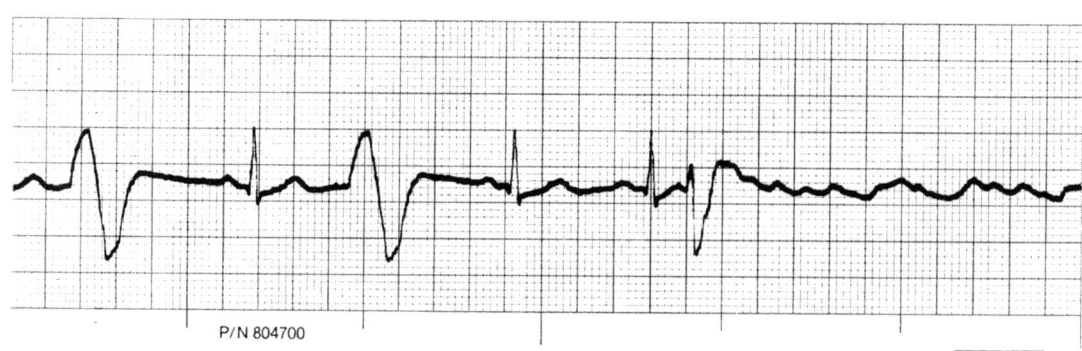

32. This patient's new EKG is:
   A. ventricular fibrillation.
   B. ventricular tachycardia.
   C. asystole.
   D. idioventricular rhythm.

33. Your first move is to:
   A. defibrillate at 200 joules.
   B. deliver a precordial thump.
   C. begin CPR.
   D. check your patient.

34. All of the following will decrease intrathoracic resistance during defibrillation EXCEPT:
   A. using electrode jelly.
   B. using proper paddle pressure.
   C. using proper paddle positioning.
   D. waiting 3–5 minutes between defibrillation attempts.

35. The preferred site for obtaining a drop of blood for glucose determination is the:
   A. fingertip.
   B. earlobe.
   C. antecubital fossa.
   D. any forearm vein.

36. Which of the following may result in a false reading?
   A. Allowing alcohol to get on the test strip.
   B. Not following the manufacturer's instructions.
   C. Touching the test strip target area.
   D. All of the above.

37. Initially, if you do not place enough blood on the test strip you should:
   A. smear it around until the target area is covered.
   B. place a second drop on top of the first.
   C. try to obtain a reading anyway.
   D. Dispose of the test strip and start over.

38. The hypoglycemic patient may present with:
  A. cool, clammy skin.
  B. altered mental status.
  C. sudden bizarre behavior.
  D. all of the above.

39. The hypoglycemic patient requires:
  A. immediate injection of insulin.
  B. immediate IV fluid boluses.
  C. immediate 50% dextrose administration.
  D. none of the above.

40. One adverse effect of administering an IV bolus medication is that it may:
  A. be slowly absorbed by the tissues.
  B. produce rapid life-threatening symptoms.
  C. be rendered inactive by the IV tubing.
  D. all of the above.

41. If, after administering 50% dextrose, your patient complains of severe pain, burning, and edema around the IV injection site, you should suspect:
  A. a pyrogenic reaction.
  B. anaphylaxis.
  C. an infiltrated IV.
  D. an outdated medication.

42. Histamine causes:
  A. bronchodilation.
  B. tissue swelling.
  C. vasoconstriction.
  D. decreased capillary permeability.

43. The person suffering from anaphylaxis presents with:
  A. wheezing.
  B. hypotension.
  C. stridor.
  D. all of the above.

44. The drug of choice for anaphylactic shock is epinephrine:
  A. 1:1000 IV.
  B. 1:1000 SC.
  C. 1:10000 SC.
  D. none of the above.

45. Epinephrine results in:
  A. bronchodilation.
  B. increased capillary permeability.
  C. vasodilation.
  D. all of the above.

46. Which of the following is true regarding subcutaneous medication injection?
  A. Fast absorption, long duration of effect.
  B. Slow absorption, long duration of effect.
  C. Fast absorption, short duration of effect.
  D. Slow absorption, short duration of effect.

47. Subcutaneous injections are given at a _____ angle.
   A. 30°
   B. 45°
   C. 60°
   D. 90°

48. Subcutaneous injections are given with a _____ gauge, _____ inch needle.
   A. 19 , 1
   B. 21 , 1/2
   C. 21 , 3/4
   D. 25 , 5/8

49. After injecting epinephrine, expect your patient's:
   A. pulse rate to fall, BP to rise.
   B. pulse rate and BP to rise.
   C. pulse rate to rise, BP to fall.
   D. pulse rate and BP to fall.

50. Absorption from an intramuscular injection occurs:
   A. immediately.
   B. within 3–5 minutes.
   C. within 10–30 minutes.
   D. none of the above.

51. Intramuscular injections are given at a _____ angle.
   A. 30°
   B. 45°
   C. 60°
   D. 90°

52. Intramuscular injections are given with a _____ gauge, _____ inch needle.
   A. 19 , 1
   B. 21 , 1/2
   C. 21 , 3/4
   D. 25 , 5/8

53. Glucagon causes which of the following actions?
   A. Converts glycogen into glucose.
   B. Releases glucose from liver.
   C. Increases in blood glucose levels.
   D. All of the above.

54. Patients with asthma and chronic obstructive pulmonary disease (COPD) may present with:
   A. dyspnea.
   B. wheezing.
   C. accessory muscle use.
   D. all of the above.

55. Advantages of using nebulized medications include:
   A. using smaller doses of the medication.
   B. rapid onset of effect.

C. limited systemic absorption.
D. all of the above.

56. When using a nebulizer, you should flow _____ liters per minute through the device.
A. 2–4
B. 4–6
C. 8–10
D. 10–15

57. Patients likely to be sent home with a Hickman in-dwelling catheter are those with:
A. cancer.
B. GI dysfunction.
C. diseases requiring long-term antibiotic therapy.
D. all of the above.

58. The Hickman is surgically placed into the:
A. right atrium.
B. left atrium.
C. right ventricle.
D. left ventricle.

59. Prehospital providers should access the Hickman:
A. routinely.
B. for fluid challenges only.
C. in life-threatening situations only.
D. none of the above.

60. Complications from accessing a Hickman in-dwelling catheter include:
A. infection.
B. air embolism.
C. damaging the catheter.
D. all of the above.

61. A pulse oximeter measures:
A. the oxygen tension in the plasma.
B. the patient's PaO_2.
C. arterial oxygen saturation.
D. venous return oxygen concentrations.

62. A normal oximeter reading is:
A. 60–100 torr.
B. 50–100%.
C. 96–100%.
D. 80–100 torr.

63. At altitudes above 5000 feet, you should expect the oximeter reading to be generally:
A. higher.
B. lower.
C. the same.
D. any of the above.

64. Situations that could falsely affect the oximeter reading include:
A. hypovolemia.
B. carbon monoxide poisoning.

C. hypothermia.
D. all of the above.

ANSWERS

1. ANS—A *IEC—312*

The great vessels enter the heart through its base. The base is the top portion of the heart located at the level of the second rib. The great vessels include the inferior and superior vena cava, aorta, pulmonary arteries, and veins.

2. ANS—B *IEC—312*

The innermost layer of the heart, which lines the chambers, is the endocardium. It is the smoothest surface known to man.

3. ANS—A *IEC—312*

The thick middle layer of the heart wall containing the bulk of the muscle mass is the myocardium. The myocardium muscle cells are unique in that they physically resemble skeletal muscles, but they have electrical properties like smooth muscle.

4. ANS—C *IEC—312*

The visceral pericardium is the layer in contact with the heart muscle itself. The outermost lining of the heart, the epicardium, is contiguous with the visceral pericardium.

5. ANS—D *IEC—312*

Surrounding the heart is a protective sac, the pericardium. The pericardium consists of two layers, the visceral pericardium and the parietal pericardium. Situated between the two layers is pericardial fluid, which acts as a lubricant during cardiac contraction.

6. ANS—C *IEC—314*

The heart contains four chambers. The two superior chambers, which receive incoming blood, are called atria. The larger inferior chambers are called ventricles.

7. ANS—D *IEC—314*

The only arteries in the body that carry oxygen-poor blood are the pulmonary arteries. These arteries carry blood from the right ventricle to the lungs for oxygenation.

8. ANS—B *IEC—314*

The only veins in the body that carry oxygen-rich blood are the pulmonary veins. These veins carry blood from the lungs back to the right atrium.

9. ANS—D *IEC—314*

The greatest muscle mass is found in the left ventricle. The left ventricle receives blood from the left atrium and pumps it out of heart into the aorta. The left side of the heart is the high-pressure side of the pump because of the high level of resistance present in the peripheral circulation.

10. ANS—B *IEC—314*

During systole the aortic and pulmonic valves are open allowing the heart to eject blood into the aorta and the pulmonary artery.

11. ANS—A *IEC—314*

During diastole, the mitral and tricuspid valves open to allow the atria to dump blood into the ventricles.

12. ANS—A *IEC—316*

The heart muscle itself is perfused by the coronary arteries. These vessels originate in the aorta just above the leaflets of the aortic valve and lie on the surface of the heart.

13. ANS—C *IEC—316*

Anastomoses between various branches of the coronary arteries allow for the development of collateral circulation. This is a protective mechanism that allows for an alternate path of blood flow in the event of vascular occlusion.

14. ANS—A *IEC—317*

Deoxygenated blood is removed from the heart through the coronary veins. The coronary veins roughly respond to the coronary arteries and drain into the right atrium.

15. ANS—C *IEC—318*

During diastole the ventricles fill with blood, the coronary arteries are perfused, and the artia contract sending blood down to the ventricles. The AV valves are open, allowing this flow of blood.

16. ANS—D *IEC—318*

Stroke volume is the amount of blood ejected by the heart in one contraction. Stroke volume is measured in milliliters. The average stroke volume is 60–100 milliliters, although this capacity can increase significantly in a healthy heart.

17. ANS—A *IEC—318*

The pressure in the ventricle at the end diastole is referred to as preload. Preload influences the force of the next contraction. This is based on Starling's Law of the Heart, which states that the more the myocardial muscle is stretched, up to a limit, the greater its force of contraction will be.

18. ANS—A *IEC—318*

Cardiac output is defined as the volume of blood pumped by the heart in one minute. It is a calculation of stroke volume times heart rate. A person with a stroke volume of 70 milliliters and heart rate of 80 beats per minute has a cardiac output therefore of 5600 milliliters.

19. ANS—C *IEC—324*

Within the cardiac muscle fibers are special structures called intercalated disks. These disks connect cardiac muscle fibers and conduct electrical impulses quickly from one muscle fiber to the next.

20. ANS—A *IEC—324*

A syncytium is a group of cardiac muscle cells that physiologically function as a unit. The ventricular syncytium occurs in an inferior to superior direction in order to direct blood flow to the aorta and the pulmonary artery.

21. ANS—C *IEC—324*

The normal intrinsic firing rate of the SA node is 60–100 beats per minute.

22. ANS—B *IEC—324*

The normal intrinsic firing rate of the AV junction is 40–60 beats per minute.

23. ANS—A *IEC—324*

The normal intrinsic firing rate of the purkinje system is 20–40 beats per minute.

24. ANS—D *IEC—326*

Only a very limited amount of information can be obtained from a single-lead ECG reading. You can tell how fast the heart is beating, how regular the heart beat is, and how long it takes to conduct the impulse through various parts of the heart. You cannot tell the presence or location of an infarct, chamber enlargement, or the quality or presence of pumping action.

25. ANS—A *IEC—327*

On the vertical axis of the standard ECG graph paper, a deflection of two large boxes signifies one millivolt of amplitude.

26. ANS—C *IEC—327*

On the horizontal axis of the standard ECG graph paper, a deflection of one large box signifies 0.2 seconds duration.

27. ANS—A *IEC—331*

The P wave represents each atrial depolarization.

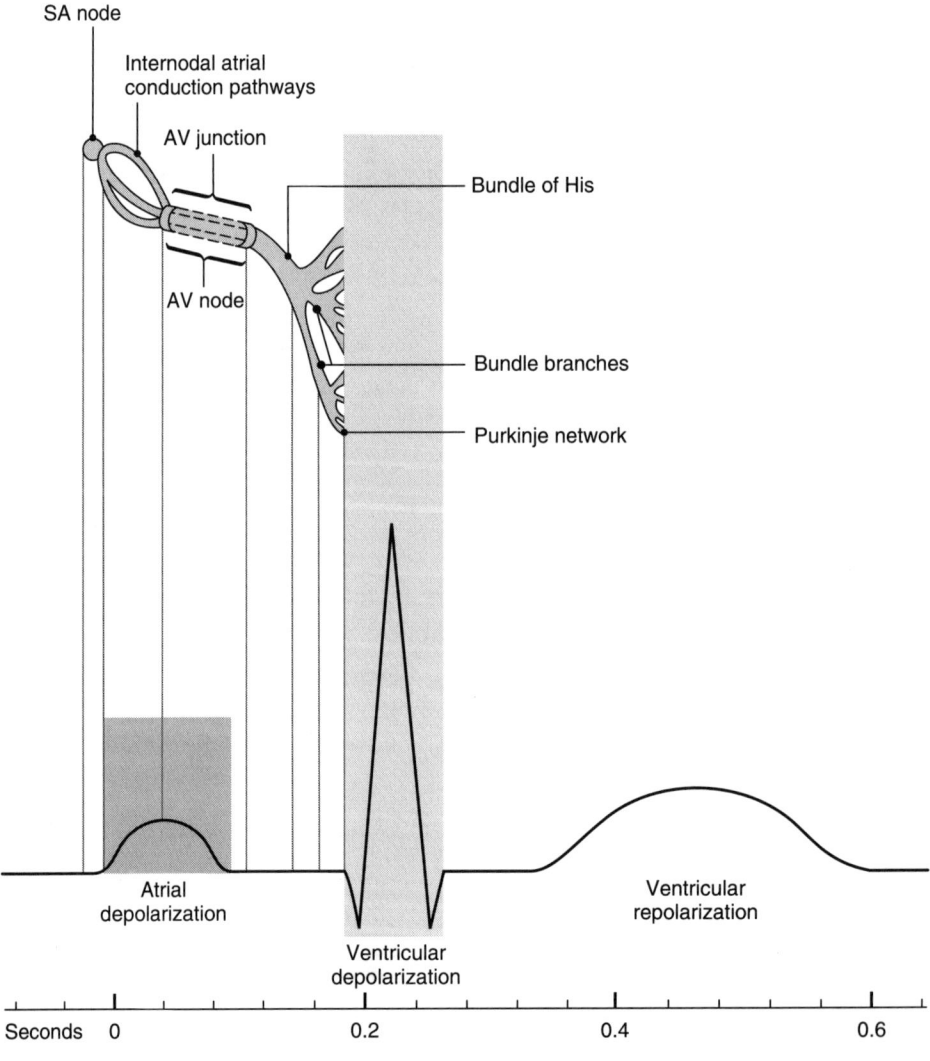

28. ANS—D *IEC—331*

The T wave represents ventricular repolarization.

Appendix **77**

29. ANS—B *IEC—331*

The QRS complex represents ventricular depolarization.

30. ANS—C *IEC—334*

The P-R interval represents delay at the AV node. The normal P-R interval is 0.12–0.20 seconds.

31. ANS—D *IEC—330*

Artifacts are deflections produced by factors other than the heart's electrical activity. Common causes of artifacts include muscle tremors, shivering, patient movement, loose electrodes, 60 Hz interference, and machine malfunction.

32. ANS—A *IEC—335*

Ventricular fibrillation is a chaotic ventricular rhythm usually resulting from the presence of many re-entry circuits within the ventricles. There is no ventricular depolarization or contraction.

33. ANS—D *IEC—338*

The initial management of this patient is to check him clinically. Always correlate your patient's pulse with what you see on the ECG. In this case, a disconnected lead or faulty monitor could produce this ECG pattern. If you cannot detect a pulse, consider the rhythm ventricular fibrillation.

34. ANS—D *IEC—340*

Reducing intrathoracic resistance is an important factor in a successful defibrillation. Using electrode jelly, proper paddle positioning and pressure, and delivering successive countershocks as quickly as possible will all decrease intrathoracic resistance.

35. ANS—A *IEC—347*

The tip of the finger is the preferred site for performing a blood glucose determination.

36. ANS—D *IEC—347*

When using any device to test a patient's blood sugar, it is important to follow the manufacturer's instructions carefully. Always calibrate the machine and match the code numbers on the test strip bottle and the machine readout. Never use outdated test strips. When using the strips, don't allow alcohol to touch the target area and never place a second drop of blood onto the strip.

37. ANS—D *IEC—347*

If you fail to adequately cover the target area with a single drop of blood, do not attempt to smear it over the area or to allow a second drop to hit the area. Simply discard the test strip and start over.

38. ANS—D *IEC—353*

The hypoglycemic patient may present with an altered mental status from the lack of glucose for brain function; cool, clammy skin and tachycardia from sympathetic nervous system stimulation; a sudden onset of bizarre or combative behavior; or coma.

39 ANS—C *IEC—353*

The brain demands a constant supply of glucose and oxygen. If left without either, the brain cells will die. Administer 50% glucose immediately to any patient with a documented hypoglycemia.

40. ANS—B *IEC—360*

Since you are delivering medications directly into the circulatory system, complications will occur rapidly and may be life-threatening.

41. ANS—C *IEC—360*

Because 50% dextrose is very concentrated, it will cause severe irritation to surrounding tissues if the IV is not patent. The patient may complain of severe pain, burning, and edema around the injection site.

42. ANS—B *IEC—361*

During an anaphylactic reaction, histamine is released. Histamine causes bronchoconstriction, increased capillary permeability and leaking with resulting tissue edema, and vasodilation.

43. ANS—D *IEC—361*

A person suffering from anaphylaxis may present with stridor from upper airway swelling, wheezing from bronchoconstriction, and hypotension from massive vasodilation.

44. ANS—B *IEC—361*

The drug of choice for anaphylaxis is epinephrine 1:1000, 0.3–0.5 mg subcutaneously (SC). If peripheral circulation is impaired, epinephrine 1:10000 IV can be given.

45. ANS—A *IEC—361*

Epinephrine is a naturally occurring drug that causes bronchodilation, vasoconstriction, and decreases capillary permeability.

46. ANS—B *IEC—362*

When you give a drug via the subcutaneous route, initial blood concentrations of the drug will be lower. However, the drug's effects will last longer (often 20 minutes or more).

47. ANS—B *IEC—362*

Subcutaneous injections are given at a 45° angle to the skin into the fatty tissue of the upper arm, abdomen, or thigh.

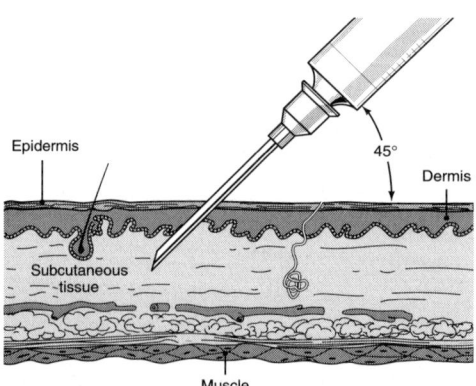

48. ANS—D *IEC—362*

Subcutaneous injections are given with a 25-gauge, 5/8-inch needle.

49. ANS—B *IEC—365*

After injecting your patient with epinephrine, expect the blood pressure and pulse rate to rise. This is due to the sympathetic nervous system stimulation.

50. ANS—C *IEC—368*

Absorption from skeletal muscle is relatively predictable. It requires approximately 10 to 30 minutes for absorption to occur.

51. ANS—D *IEC—368*

Intramuscular injections are given at a 90° angle to the skin deep into the muscle tissue, where it is absorbed by the capillaries and enters the bloodstream.

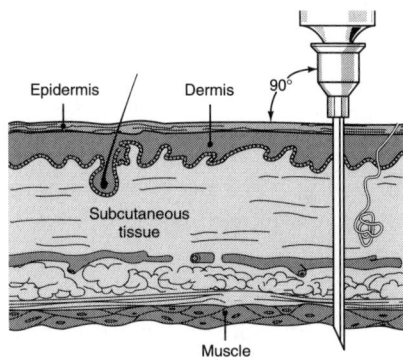

52. ANS—A *IEC—368*

Intramuscular injections are given with a 19-gauge, 1- to 1-1/2 inch needle.

53. ANS—D *IEC—367*

Glucagon is a hormone that stimulates the liver to convert glycogen stores into glucose. The liver then releases the glucose into the bloodstream for use by the body. This causes an instant elevation in blood glucose levels.

54. ANS—D *IEC—372*

Patients with airway disease such as asthma or COPD may present with marked dyspnea, wheezing, and accessory muscle use. These signs and symptoms are due to the narrowing of the lower airways making it difficult to move air in and out of the lungs.

55. ANS—D *IEC—373*

There are numerous advantages to aerosol therapy. You can use smaller doses of the drug; the effects occur rapidly because the drug is delivered directly onto the target tissues; and there is limited systemic absorption of the drug.

56. ANS—C *IEC—374*

When using a nebulizer, you should flow 8–10 liters per minute through the device.

57. ANS—D *IEC—377*

Many patients are discharged from the hospital with an indwelling catheter such as the Hickman. These are patients with cancer, debilitating illnesses, GI dysfunction, and those requiring long-term antibiotic therapy. The catheter provides instant IV access without constant venipunctures.

58. ANS—A *IEC—377*

The Hickman is surgically placed into the right atrium and protrudes from the upper chest wall.

59. ANS—C *IEC—377*

Use the Hickman catheter for life-threatening IV access only. Routine use of this site increases the risk for complications.

60. ANS—D *IEC—378*

Complications from using the Hickman catheter for IV access include air embolism, infection, and damaging the catheter during clamping procedures.

61. ANS—C *IEC—379*

The pulse oximeter determines the ratio of red blood cells that are saturated versus those that are not.

62. ANS—C *IEC—380*

A normal oximetry reading is 96–100%. A reading of 90–95% indicates a patient whose respiratory status is deteriorating. A patient with a reading <90% requires aggressive airway and ventilatory management.

63. ANS—B *IEC—383*

At altitudes above 5000 feet, the oxygen tension is reduced. As a result, oxygen is not driven into the blood as easily as at sea level. Therefore, you should expect the oximeter reading to be low.

64. ANS—D *IEC—384*

There are a number of conditions that render the pulse oximetry reading inaccurate. Carbon monoxide attaches itself more readily to the hemoglobin molecule than oxygen does. Therefore, in the case of carboxyhemoglobin, the reading will be falsely high. Low flow states in which circulation to the periphery is restricted, such as hypovolemia, hypothermia, and shock, will alter the reading. In these cases the reading will be falsely high.